Naked Truth

The Movement Against the Bra

By
Aurora M. Knight

Naked Truth

The Movement Against the Bra

Table of Contents

Introduction

The journey towards comfort and authenticity begins with a choice—a choice many women across the globe are making. That choice is to embrace bralessness, a decision that flies in the face of long-standing cultural expectations. The No-Bra Movement, burgeoning in its scope, is not just about the absence of an undergarment, but a deeper assertion of autonomy and self-definition. It represents a rejection of discomfort and societal dictation, calling into question why women have been expected to conform to certain norms for so long.

Our culture, with its vast and intricate web of expectations, has long dictated the way women should dress, act, and even present themselves. The bra, a seemingly simple piece of clothing, has been a symbol of these constraints. Whether introduced during adolescence or integrated into daily routines, they have been presented as necessary for support, modesty, and femininity. Yet, even as they were marketed for comfort, countless women have felt exactly the opposite. The No-Bra Movement raises questions about these assumptions, inviting dialogue and introspection about what women's empowerment truly looks like.

Embracing comfort doesn't merely mean reassessing what clothing we wear, but challenging the reasons behind those choices. This movement seeks to have women consider: Are we dressing for ourselves or adhering to societal pressures? It's a conversation that extends beyond the physical to touch on issues of mental and

1

emotional freedom. It shines a light on the variability of personal comfort, asking society to recognize and respect diverse definitions of femininity and self-expression.

At its core, the No-Bra Movement is inherently tied to themes of body positivity and acceptance. In a world where idealized, often unattainable beauty standards are rife, choosing to go braless is an act of defiance and self-acceptance. It reclaims the narrative around a woman's body, promoting the idea that beauty is individual and does not need to be molded by the designs of external forces. By challenging the traditional standards of beauty, the movement pushes back against objectification, advocating for a woman's right to define herself on her own terms.

For some, the journey towards rejecting the bra might seem daunting, particularly given the cultural and societal pushback. In numerous cultures, bras are more than just underpieces of clothing; they are seen as markers of propriety and civility. Yet, this movement emboldens individuals to overcome the fear of judgment and aim for personal comfort. It's about creating spaces where women can decide for themselves what brings them comfort without feeling subjected to external scrutiny.

One might wonder, how did we arrive at a point where such a simple decision requires advocacy and social catalysts? To understand this, we must consider the historical and sociopolitical layers that surround the bra. Originally designed as a functional garment, it gradually became entangled with notions of female propriety and social status. The movement towards discarding bras is thus a continuation of a larger dialogue about women's rights and autonomy, reminiscent of past feminist waves that sought to dismantle gender norms and empower women.

Empowerment, in this context, is multifaceted, involving not just the removal of a piece of clothing, but the broader conceptualization of freedom. It's about women having the ability to choose for themselves, free from guilt or obligation, and to inhabit spaces where their decisions are theirs alone. This movement isn't prescriptive—it acknowledges the spectrum of comfort and leaves room for individual differences, recognizing that empowerment means different things to different people.

As the dialogue about embracing or rejecting bras continues to grow, it serves as an inspiration for other movements centered on body autonomy. It is a testament to the power of community, solidarity, and activism to spark change and challenge age-old paradigms. The stories emerging from this movement are rich and varied, each illustrating the personal victories and challenges faced by those who dare to venture into uncharted territory.

These stories, whether they arise from public figures using their platforms to endorse body autonomy or everyday individuals sharing their journeys on social media, underscore the pervasive nature of this dialogue. They reflect a world inching towards inclusivity and understanding. And while the movement's journey is far from complete, it has set in motion the gears of change, pointing towards a future where personal comfort takes precedence over societal expectations.

In examining the No-Bra Movement, it is easy to see it as a microcosm of larger ongoing societal shifts. The themes it encapsulates resonate with ongoing struggles for gender equality, redefining femininity, and the quest for personal authenticity. Through embracing change, we find the courage to reinterpret established norms and foster newer, more inclusive avenues for expression and identity.

This book delves into the heart of the No-Bra Movement, drawing on rich cultural, historical, and personal contexts. Its aim is to inform, inspire, and empower readers by highlighting the significance of choosing comfort and authenticity in a world that often demands conformity. By sharing stories, perspectives, and insights, we hope to illuminate the paths trodden by those who've ventured boldly into the realms of self-definition and autonomy.

Let this be a testament to the resilience and courage of those who choose to challenge convention, offering a glimpse into a future where everyone can exist comfortably, free of unnecessary constraints.

Chapter 1:
The History of the Bra

The evolution of the bra is a fascinating journey that highlights women's relentless pursuit of comfort and autonomy. Emerging from rudimentary garments designed to bind and conceal, the bra has evolved into a multifaceted symbol of both support and societal expectation. This cultural artifact, rooted as far back as ancient civilizations who crafted simple forms of breast support with natural materials, has seen dramatic transformations over the centuries. The 20th century marked a pivotal era, with rapid commercial growth and technological advancements that paved the way for today's diverse offerings. Bras have transcended their utilitarian roots to become instruments of personal expression, reflecting broader social changes and a growing emphasis on empowerment and choice. Across different eras, each design shift tells a story of women's ongoing negotiation with body image, freedom, and societal norms, setting the stage for the more recent movements advocating for comfort and rejecting constraints. This historical trajectory sets a foundation for understanding why the conversation around bras remains vibrant and essential to the broader discourse on women's rights and body autonomy.

Early Developments in Bra Design

The history of the bra is marked by a fascinating journey from rudimentary attempts at breast support to the intricate designs of today. In the early stages of this story, we witness a mixture of necessity and innovation. Women have always sought ways to manage their bodies in a way that aligns with their needs and societal expectations. The impulse to create a garment that both supports and enhances dates back centuries, driven by a blend of function and fashion.

The earliest garments that can be considered precursors to the bra were not merely about modesty or aesthetics; they had a distinctly practical function. In ancient Greece, women wrapped bands of wool or linen around their bodies under the bust to lift and support their breasts. This primitive design was called the *apodesmos*, or *strophion*. Its simplicity and effectiveness underscore a fundamental desire for comfort and support, an echo that resonates throughout the history of bra design.

During the Roman era, there was a shift toward more structured clothing, which included the use of the *strophium* or *mamillare*. These were bands tied around the breasts, achieving a flattening effect that emphasized a lean silhouette favored by Roman style ideals. Fashion, in this era, started to influence design choices, intertwining practicality with aesthetic results. However, the lack of customization in these early examples meant that comfort was often sacrificed for the sake of adhering to fashion's whims.

Fast forward to the Middle Ages, and we find that constraints tightened even more. Corsets, a dominant force in women's fashion, started to replace earlier, simpler methods of breast support. These devices were designed to reshape the body, often to extremes, by constricting and flattening the chest as part of creating an exaggerated hourglass figure. Comfort once again took a backseat, as societal norms dictated rigid compliance with fashionable silhouettes.

The 19th century marked a turning point, a prelude to modernity in bra design. As the industrial revolution spurred advancements in production and materials, the need for more practical undergarments finally took precedence. Women, increasingly involved in public and professional life, demanded clothing that supported their activities. This period observed the gradual decline of the oppressive corset, paving the way for more humane alternatives.

Several inventors began experimenting with designs that liberated the body while providing necessary support. One of the first recorded patents for a modern bra-like garment was filed in 1869 by a Frenchman named Herminie Cadolle, who created the "corselet gorge," which separated the corset into two pieces, liberating the bust. However, it took nearly half a century before Cadolle's vision significantly impacted mainstream fashion.

In 1914, the brassiere as we know it took a notable leap forward thanks to Mary Phelps Jacob. Tired of the restrictive corsets, she designed a soft, backless bra from silk handkerchiefs and ribbon, creating a rudimentary yet groundbreaking design. Jacob's innovation, later patented as the "Backless Brassiere," set the stage for the bras of the future—a garment driven by both comfort and functionality.

As women's roles in society evolved, so too did the expectations for their clothing. The suffrage movement and women's participation in the workforce during World War I catalyzed a seismic shift in attitudes towards undergarments. The thirst for liberation from outdated styles meant that designs now needed to meet functional, rather than purely ornamental, standards. This popularized Jacob's bra design and 'freer' undergarments began to take the place of the Victorian corset.

The 1920s, often remembered for the flapper era, saw a rejection of the traditional curves that corsets accentuated. Flappers preferred a more androgynous silhouette, which translated into less structured lingerie. The bandeau bra came into vogue—a simple band that offered a minimalistic approach to breast support. This choice symbolized a radical shift towards personal freedom and a sociocultural transformation in how women's bodies were perceived and adorned.

The following decades ushered in numerous developments that refined the design and function of bras. The advent of elasticated materials in the 1930s allowed for better fit and comfort, aligning the garment with the modern woman's multifaceted lifestyle. By the 1950s, the bullet bra became iconic, emphasizing a pointed shape popularized by silver screen sirens, illustrating how bras had become instruments of fashion and identity.

Through these iterations, one thing remained constant: the search for a balance between comfort and societal expectations. Innovators and designers continue to build on the foundation laid by early developments, striving to reconcile the often opposing forces of comfort, style, and societal norms. Each epoch of bra design reflects broader changes in women's roles, rights, and self-expression, charting a path from constraint to liberation.

In tracing the evolution of bra design, we find a narrative both of constraint and breakthrough. Today, as discussions around body positivity and autonomy gather momentum, the bra's early history invites us to reconsider how garments can empower rather than restrict. Past lessons drive the movement towards designs that honor both body and spirit, advocating for freedom that respects the individual's choices.

The Rise of the Bra Industry

The bra industry as we know it didn't develop overnight. Its rise was a complex dance of cultural shifts, technological advancements, and social demands. It emerged during a time when women's roles were being redefined, yet their bodies were still seen as objects to be molded and controlled. The early 20th century marked the beginning of a significant transformation in how intimate apparel was produced and marketed, driven largely by the industrial revolution and wartime necessities.

In the years leading up to World War I, women were beginning to experience unprecedented shifts in societal roles. The suffragette movement was gaining momentum, and women were slowly entering the workforce. Corsets, which had been the standard for centuries, were becoming impractical. The need for more comfortable, less restrictive undergarments catalyzed the birth of the bra industry. Many women were drawn to the promise of the brassiere—a garment that offered support without the rigidity of a corset.

The war itself acted as a catalyst for industrial growth. With men fighting, women took up jobs in factories, necessitating more sensible clothing options. This demand was met by innovators who saw the potential for profit in creating undergarments that aligned with these new realities. The production techniques developed during wartime enabled manufacturers to mass-produce bras, significantly reducing costs and making them accessible to a wider demographic.

By the 1920s, the bra had begun to step out of the shadows as a mere undergarment to become a symbol of fashion and status. Advertisers and designers played a pivotal role in transforming public perception of bras from practical items to essential components of a woman's wardrobe. They tapped into the societal desire for freedom and modernity, showcasing bras in fashion magazines, department store windows, and even on the silver screen. These marketing efforts did more than just sell bras; they shaped an entire industry that prized innovation and consumerism.

Fast forward to the mid-20th century, and the industry had grown into a powerful force. The 1950s introduced bullet bras and push-up styles that promised an idealized feminine silhouette. Television and movies idolized women whose figures were accentuated by these designs, thereby creating a cultural obsession with the hourglass shape.

Companies thrived by perpetually adapting to fashion trends and consumer desires, ensuring their products were indispensable.

The bra industry didn't just thrive on its product innovation—it also capitalized on the intersection of comfort and fashion. As fabric technology advanced, so did the variety of bras available. Cotton and nylon were woven into more elastic and comfortable designs, allowing manufacturers to appeal to the sensibility of the modern woman. Still, this melding of function and fashion often prioritized aesthetic appearance over genuine comfort.

In the 1970s, as societal norms began to shift once more toward liberation and self-expression, the bra industry was forced to adapt. The women's liberation movement challenged long-held beliefs about female appearances and comfort. Bras became a symbol of conformity and repression for some, leading to public demonstrations where they were sometimes burned in protest. The industry responded by diversifying its offerings and marketing campaigns to include designs that promised freedom and individuality.

Throughout the late 20th century and into the new millennium, the bra industry rode the waves of cultural change with remarkable agility. It leveraged advances in digital marketing and social media to remain relevant and desirable. New brands emerged with a focus on inclusivity, offering a broader range of sizes and styles that catered to a more diverse consumer base. Still, for all its adaptations, the industry consistently found ways to balance the scales between fashion-forward and function-focused designs.

Today, the bra industry stands at a unique crossroads. It faces a consumer base that's more informed and vocal about their needs and discomforts than ever before. As the no-bra movement garners attention, traditional manufacturers are beginning to reconsider what true innovation means—shifting away from pushing ostensibly perfect bodies toward designing for authenticity and comfort. This evolving landscape presents both a challenge and an opportunity for the industry to redefine its relationship with those it serves.

As the bra industry continues to evolve, its trajectory offers keen insights into broader societal values and transitions. It not only reflects changes in women's fashion but also embodies the ongoing dialogue about women's rights, autonomy, and comfort. This industry, while steeped in commercial interests, mirrors the cultural battles fought over how women choose to present and perceive themselves. In understanding its history, we glean lessons on resilience, adaptation, and the enduring quest for personal freedom.

Chapter 2:
The Origins of the No-Bra Movement

The origins of the No-Bra Movement mark a pivotal shift in the narrative of women's self-expression, demanding a dialogue on bodily comfort that challenges conventional restraints. Spurred partially by the discomfort of traditional garments, the movement's early advocates viewed bras as symbols of societal expectations and limitations on female autonomy. Rooted in the broader waves of feminism, this liberation wasn't solely about an article of clothing; it was a stand against the imposition of conformist beauty and comfort standards. As women began to push back against these norms, a new path was forged—one where women claimed the right to decide their own comfort, free from the historical baggage that dictated their choices. This burgeoning sense of empowerment fueled a collective desire to redefine femininity on their own terms, pioneering a movement that transcends mere rebellion and blossoms into a celebration of authenticity and personal freedom.

Early Advocates for Comfort

The journey towards comfort wasn't a sprint, but rather a steady progression marked by individual acts of defiance and quiet rebellion. Early advocates for comfort in the no-bra movement, although perhaps not fully aware of the cultural revolution they were igniting, began to question the societal norms that dictated women's attire. These pioneers—women who chose comfort over convention—broke away from the rigid expectations of what it meant to be feminine and embraced a sense of bodily autonomy. Their stories resonate, even today, as whispers of courage that speak volumes.

It often started with small, personal decisions to forgo bras, driven by the sheer desire for comfort and authenticity. These women demonstrated that confidence and femininity weren't tethered to constrictive clothing. Each step they took towards comfort, sometimes quite literally, was an affirmation of their right to make choices about their bodies. These advocates set the stage for discussions that challenged the status quo.

Many early trailblazers in this movement did not engage in organized activism. Rather, their influence stemmed from personal actions that inspired others. Feminists of the 1960s and 70s are often credited with popularizing no-bra living as part of the broader women's liberation movement. However, the seeds of this change were planted much earlier by women who dared to live by their own rules. These pioneers sometimes emerged from diverse backgrounds, yet shared a common thread of seeking liberation from the unnecessary constraints of structured undergarments.

Among those who questioned the necessity of the bra were women from artistic communities who found the traditional attire not just uncomfortable, but also creatively stifling. These early adopters often faced criticism and even ridicule, as societal expectations weighed heavily against their choices. They didn't see their chests as something to be hidden or molded into preconceived notions of beauty. Rather, they embraced natural shapes, finding empowerment in authenticity.

Cultural shifts are often marked by the visionaries who see the world not as it is, but as it could be. These women were no different. Advocates for comfort served as living examples that rejecting the conventional could coexist with grace and strength. In resisting the era's traditional norms, they paved the way for a dialogue about personal freedom and bodily autonomy—conversations critical to the ongoing fight for gender equality.

One remarkable aspect was how these advocates found ways to subtly educate and encourage others, sparking important conversations without the benefit of contemporary platforms like social media. The early movement relied on word-of-mouth and grassroots sharing. News of their choices spread through communities, slowly chipping away at the prevailing myth that bras were non-negotiable for proper womanhood.

These women stood as quiet beacons of change and laid the groundwork for future movements. They taught us that choosing comfort wasn't shirking tradition, but rather, reframing what tradition could mean. They didn't see rebellion as a loud proclamation, but as a personal declaration of independence that spoke through their everyday lives. Their legacy continues to inspire an ever-growing number of individuals to re-examine their own relationships with clothing, comfort, and personal identity.

The experiences of early advocates serve as poignant reminders of the power of individual choice in challenging societal norms. They gave others permission to explore and prioritize comfort. In a world still grappling with rigid standards of femininity, their actions were and are invaluable. By navigating a path less trodden, these women incrementally prompted broader cultural shifts, ushering in an era that increasingly values personal well-being over conformity.

The Role of Feminism in the Movement

Understanding the no-bra movement requires dissecting the profound influence that feminism has played in its development. Feminism, with its core mission to advocate for equality and autonomy, naturally intersects with the ideals of the no-bra movement. At its heart, feminism seeks to dismantle societal structures that dictate how women should present themselves, and freeing oneself from the bra is a literal and metaphorical shedding of these constraining norms. This isn't just about comfort; it's about reclaiming agency over one's own body.

Consider the social climate from which the no-bra movement emerged. During the height of second-wave feminism in the 1960s and 70s, women began publicly challenging traditional gender roles and the expectations that came with them. The bra, often seen as a symbol of these restrictive expectations, naturally became a target. To many feminists, bras represented a social mandate for women to conform to a particular mold—one that was not only physically uncomfortable but also psychologically confining.

Feminism offered the ideological groundwork necessary for questioning why women were expected to wear bras in the first place. It urged women to scrutinize the arbitrariness of social norms that dictated intimate aspects of their lives. The liberation from bras was not just about ending discomfort but also about rejecting the idea that women's bodies must fit into a certain shape or be policed by societal standards. This act of rebellion resonated with feminists who were already questioning various other aspects of gender inequality.

What's poignant about the role of feminism in the no-bra movement is how it seamlessly weaves together issues of body autonomy and self-definition with broader social justice themes. For feminists, the movement highlighted a critical site of struggle—how women's bodies were spaces of control and commodification. Going braless was a powerful statement that counteracted not just fashion industry pressures but also patriarchal assumptions about modesty and propriety.

Notably, feminist theorists emphasized that the decision to wear or not wear a bra should be up to the individual and free from judgment. This emphasis on choice was radical in an era where expectations of femininity often left little room for personal autonomy. Feminism, therefore, provided both the critical framework and the moral support for countless women to question, choose, and act in accordance with their comfort and values.

While the movement's early stages were deeply entwined with feminist actions and protests, it's important to note that the narrative has evolved. The feminist aspects of the no-bra movement have been sustained and redefined by subsequent generations, from third-wave feminists in the 1990s to present-day activists. For contemporary feminists, going braless often connects with larger conversations about inclusivity and intersectionality—ensuring that the movement recognizes the diverse experiences of all women.

For instance, third-wave feminism, with its embrace of diversity, expanded the conversation to include women of different races, body types, and socioeconomic statuses who might experience the no-bra movement differently. These conversations have only grown more nuanced, influenced by global feminist discourses that highlight how cultural contexts affect women's choices around their bodies. Feminism has propelled the no-bra movement into a more complex landscape where personal agency and cultural influences intersect uniquely.

Moreover, the feminist discourse surrounding the no-bra movement isn't limited to women but also engages men. Feminist ideology argues for societal recognition of gender equality, including the elimination of gender-specific pressures. By questioning why women's dress and comfort choices are scrutinized more harshly than men's, the movement invites broader discussions of gender norms and the implicit power dynamics they perpetuate.

The internet, and particularly social media, have also amplified feminist voices within the no-bra movement. Digital platforms provide spaces for discourse, advocacy, and community building. Here, feminist ideology aids in dismantling ongoing societal myths about femininity, allowing for greater solidarity and shared narrative creation. The connectedness of these platforms also ensures that the movement remains fluid and open to new interpretations and challenges.

At its core, feminism in the no-bra movement demands a radical reimagining of comfort and autonomy. It demands that society reflects on the internalized norms that dictate why bras are worn and why going without one can be seen as subversive. It demands a broader context where all bodily choices are respected and validated. The feminist legacy within the movement is one of questioning and challenging, ensuring that the movement continues to evolve and adapt to the changing landscape of women's rights and social expectations.

In summary, the role of feminism in the no-bra movement is both foundational and transformative, deeply entwined with the ongoing fight for women's rights and body positivity. By challenging norms and advocating for autonomy, feminism has not only spearheaded the movement's growth but also secured its relevance in today's pursuit of comfort and self-expression. As feminism continues to evolve, so too will the no-bra movement, rooted in the timeless quest for personal freedom and societal equality.

Chapter 3:
Health Implications of Wearing Bras

The health implications of wearing bras have long been a topic of debate, stirring passionate discussions about body autonomy and the intersection of comfort and societal expectations. While some argue that bras offer necessary support and potentially reduce back pain, others caution against their possible impact on natural lymph circulation and question their contribution to breast sagging over time. Scientific studies present mixed results, challenging the notion of bras as either essential or detrimental, and highlighting the need for more comprehensive research. In this context, many women are reevaluating their relationship with bras, empowered by a growing awareness of personal comfort and health. This nuanced dialogue invites a broader exploration of how individual choices can redefine our understanding of self-care, underscoring the importance of listening to one's body and embracing comfort without compromise.

The Debate on Breast Health

In the ongoing conversation about bras and breast health, divergent views swirl around with fervor. For many, the bra is seen as more than just an item of clothing; it's a symbol of societal expectations, comfort, and potentially, controversy regarding health. Proponents of bras argue they're essential for support and preventing breast sagging. Meanwhile, detractors question their health benefits, challenging the notion with both scientific studies and personal anecdotes.

For some time, the medical community has been engaged in examining the potential health implications of wearing bras. The traditional standpoint suggests that bras help prevent the stretching of breast tissue by providing much-needed support, especially for women with larger breasts. This viewpoint is heavily marketed by the bra industry, which capitalizes on the fear of sagging—the ultimate, but perhaps overblown, menace to youthful looks and female desirability. Yet, this assumption, steadfast as it may be, rests on controversial scientific ground.

Skeptics of the necessity of bras point to studies that either refute or show nuanced results regarding their benefits. Some researchers suggest that wearing bras might impair circulation, potentially affecting lymphatic drainage. Impaired drainage can theoretically lead to the buildup of toxins, raising questions about long-term breast health. However, it's crucial to note that evidence on this front remains inconclusive, leaving plenty of room for individual interpretation and choice.

A watershed moment came from a study in France conducted by sports scientist Jean-Denis Rouillon. His research, although limited in scope, challenged conventional wisdom. Rouillon proposed that bras might actually be counterproductive, leading to weaker, less-structured breast tissue over time. His findings ignited both criticism and intrigue, feeding the fire of a debate that's as much about personal experience as it is about scientific discovery.

This debate taps into broader issues of autonomy. For many women, wearing a bra isn't just a question of physical comfort; it's deeply tied to personal freedom and self-expression. Shouldn't each woman have the right to choose what's best for her body without feeling the weight of societal judgement? This very question fuels the no-bra movement as a pivotal subsect of the broader body positivity and women's rights movements. Challenges to the notion of "obligatory bra-wearing" are raising questions about traditional beauty standards and encouraging a re-evaluation of comfort over conformity.

Yet, it's important to recognize that the choice to wear or forgo a bra isn't just an abstract debate. For some, the very design of bras can lead to discomfort, creating issues ranging from skin irritation to back and shoulder pain caused by ill-fitting straps and underwires. In these cases, not wearing a bra can be a pragmatic choice for health and well-being. On the flip side, some women feel empowered and supported by bras, appreciating the lifted, polished look and the confidence it brings in professional and social settings.

The conversation around breast health and bras leans heavily on individual context. Everyone's anatomy is different. Some prefer the added layer of support, while others revel in the freedom of bralessness. This diversity opines that one-size-fits-all advice is rarely appropriate. The conversation about bras becomes even more nuanced when discussing age, pregnancy, and postpartum conditions, all of which can alter breast shape and the need for support.

Beyond personal choice, commercial implications amplify the debate on breast health. The bra industry is a multi-billion-dollar behemoth that plays a significant role in social narratives about femininity and beauty. Its marketing prowess shapes public perceptions of what is "normal" or "beautiful" for women, often pushing consumers away from considering alternative perspectives.

However, there's a burgeoning awareness that bra-wearing is not strictly about health or aesthetics. It's part of a larger cultural discourse about body autonomy—an acknowledgment that our bodies are our own to adorn or leave bare as we see fit. This realization is freeing for many, aligning with broader movements that champion women's rights and the collapsing of rigid gender norms.

In this era of widespread connectivity, discussions on breast health and bras proliferate across forums and social media platforms, empowering individuals with access to a multitude of perspectives. These open dialogues challenge myths and breed understanding, allowing for the celebration of diverse experiences in women's lives. With more voices rising to share personal narratives, the discussion around bras and breast health continues to evolve into a realm of informed personal choice rather than prescriptive norm.

As the dialogue progresses, the notion that "comfort" may transcend its traditional associations, extending into an untapped realm of psychological well-being, begins to take shape. The decision, whether to wear a bra or not, can resonate deeply with individual comfort levels—both physically and mentally. This choice embodies a significant personal narrative for many women, granting them a sense of control amid the cacophony of societal expectations.

The interplay between bras, breast health, and personal choice signifies an ongoing journey toward empowerment and autonomy. By engaging in this debate, women are continually redefining their own experiences, shifting the paradigm from a health concern to an embodiment of identity and choice. The lenses through which we view bras and breast health shouldn't be static but adaptive, receptive, and inclusive of all women's voices, paving the way for broader acceptance and understanding.

Studies and Scientific Perspectives

When it comes to the centuries-old tradition of wearing bras, discussions often pivot to their health implications. As societal norms evolve, so does scientific inquiry, which seeks to dissect the potentially beneficial and detrimental effects of bras on women's health. Studies and scientific perspectives provide a diverse array of insights, challenging preconceived notions and offering a deeper understanding of this everyday garment.

Over the years, researchers have engaged with the complex relationship between bras and breast health, often with polarizing results. Some studies suggest that wearing bras excessively might impede the natural movement of breast tissue, potentially affecting circulation and lymphatic flow. This notion stems from a theory proposed by a few researchers that highlights the importance of allowing natural tissue movement for breast health maintenance. However, it's imperative to note that this hypothesis hasn't gained unanimous support across the scientific community.

On the flip side, many experts argue in favor of bras, emphasizing their role in providing support, reducing breast movement during physical activity, and therefore helping to prevent discomfort or injury. A significant number of studies back the claim that bras, particularly sports bras, can alleviate stress on the skin and underlying tissues during exercise, highlighting their importance for active lifestyles. The argument revolves around the practical benefits rather than health detriments, showcasing how varied and context-dependent the science can be.

Further complicating the issue is the topic of breast sagging, medically referred to as ptosis. The debate about whether wearing a bra can prevent sagging has been ongoing. Some contend that constant breast support might lead the tissue to become reliant on the external support, possibly weakening the ligaments over time. In contrast, traditional views endorse bras as a method to maintain breast shape. Despite these discussions, the consensus remains elusive, primarily because breast sagging is influenced by numerous factors including genetics, age, and lifestyle, which are difficult to isolate in scientific studies.

Scientific inquiry has also ventured into the psychological realm, examining how bras impact women's mental well-being. For some women, the act of wearing a bra is associated with adherence to societal norms and expectations, which can cause discomfort or stress. Understanding the psychological comfort and confidence associated with opting out of wearing a bra is an ongoing area of research. The liberation from such constraints can have profound implications for mental health, a perspective growing in recognition among health professionals.

Adding another dimension to this multifaceted subject are studies exploring the long-term health implications of bra-wearing habits. This includes the examination of potential links between bra use and issues such as back pain, shoulder strain, and even breast cancer. While early hypotheses suggested a correlation between tight bras and an increased cancer risk, later studies have generally debunked that myth, illustrating the importance of evidence-based understanding over anecdotal fears.

Moreover, biomechanical studies present an emerging field exploring how different designs and materials impact breast support and comfort. These analyses contribute to the development of bras that can better accommodate diverse body types and breast sizes, aiming to optimize both health and comfort. Engineers and health scientists are keenly interested in advancing bra technology, ensuring that new designs do not compromise body autonomy for the sake of aesthetics or tradition.

Importantly, the methodology of prior studies often comes under scrutiny. The lack of large-scale, long-term studies and reliance on self-reported data compound the difficulty in deriving definitive conclusions. However, contemporary scientists are increasingly focusing on longitudinal research, which could illuminate long-standing questions with more clarity.

As scientific exploration continues, collaboration across disciplines becomes crucial. Health professionals, sociologists, and designers are working together to foster a comprehensive understanding, placing women's comfort and health at the forefront. This intersectional approach recognizes the multifarious factors influencing individual choices and societal trends regarding bras.

In summary, while the scientific community has made significant strides in exploring the health implications of wearing bras, much remains to be understood. The varying viewpoints and ongoing debates exemplify the complexity of the issue, encouraging further research. Scientific perspectives, armed with empiricism and modern methodologies, continue to evolve, motivating a more informed dialogue. As society progresses towards greater body autonomy and empowerment, these studies play a pivotal role in guiding informed personal choices and challenging societal norms.

Chapter 4:
Social Perspectives on
the No-Bra Trend

The no-bra trend has ignited a powerful dialogue across diverse social landscapes, challenging entrenched norms about gender roles and comfort. As more women choose to forgo traditional bras, society's reactions have ranged from encouragement to resistance. This shift disrupts conventional markers of femininity, prompting conversations about the essence of comfort and autonomy in a gendered world. For many, it's an act of liberation, an opportunity to reclaim bodily agency in a space long dominated by prescriptive attire. While some perceive the trend as emblematic of broader feminist gains, others grapple with its implications on public decorum and identity. Yet, underlying these discussions is a common thread: a reevaluation of what it means to be comfortable in one's own skin, sparking aspirations for a more inclusive understanding of personal freedom. Embracing such change isn't merely about rejecting a garment; it's about embracing diverse expressions of self and advocating for a future where everyone's comfort holds equal importance.

Society's Reaction to Change

The no-bra trend, ever since its rise, has been like a pebble tossed into the waters of societal norms, creating ripples of reactions that range from enthusiastic support to staunch criticism. Initially, it seemed to challenge the deeply rooted fashion and social conventions which had dictated women's clothing choices for centuries. The allure of comfort, liberation from binding garments, and an embrace of body positivity stirred a diverse set of responses. Often, society struggles with change, especially when it involves questioning traditional values. This has certainly been the case with the no-bra movement, which, in its bold confrontation with status quo, epitomizes the turmoil that accompanies any significant cultural shift.

For many supporters, the no-bra trend represents a step toward autonomy, allowing women to make choices based solely on their comfort rather than societal expectations. It empowers individuals to embrace their natural form, which resonates with various feminist ideologies. These proponents argue that the expectation for women to wear bras is yet another method of enforcing control over women's bodies. The movement, therefore, is seen as a liberating act—a march toward equality where women are granted the freedom to choose what makes them comfortable. Social media has played a massive role in galvanizing support, with online communities forming to share stories, encouragement, and advice.

However, not everyone has welcomed this change with open arms. Traditionalists and certain segments of the population perceive the no-bra trend as a challenge to decorum and modesty. For them, bras are synonymous with professionalism and neatness, reflecting a belief that without one, women might appear unkempt or improperly bold. This perspective often spills over into workplace dynamics, impacting dress codes and presenting potential conflicts. In this light, the no-bra trend collides with an ingrained societal norm that equates a woman's respectability with her adherence to certain dress protocols.

Though divisive, the debate over bralessness has fostered essential discussions about gender norms and the historical policing of women's bodies. It has highlighted an inconsistency in societal expectations—

why should clothing comfort be more accessible to one gender over another? Men have enjoyed the luxury of dressing without restrictions traditionally, while women have long endured exacting standards. The clash of opinions around the no-bra movement brings this discrepancy into sharp relief, questioning outdated norms and advocating for a more inclusive understanding of dress and comfort.

Interestingly, across different cultures, the reactions vary, emphasizing local customs and historical attitudes toward women's clothing. Some societies, more accustomed to relaxed dress codes, have embraced the no-bra movement with little controversy, seeing it as a natural progression toward personal freedom. Others, steeped in more conservative traditions, struggle with this loosening of sartorial expectations, viewing it as a rebellion against cultural values. This global variance underscores the broader cultural dialogue that the no-bra trend has instigated, challenging communities worldwide to consider their own preconceived notions about femininity and sexuality.

Beyond cultural and traditional boundaries, age and generational gaps also account for differing perceptions of the no-bra trend. Younger generations, often more attuned to progressive changes, generally express greater acceptance and curiosity, seeing it as part of broader socio-cultural shifts. Older generations, who may have experienced the rigidity of past fashion norms firsthand, sometimes view the movement with skepticism or caution. This generational divide hints at evolving views on gender roles and provides a lens into how societal progress is often a generational relay, passed and adapted over time.

Narratives around modesty and professionalism have often served as barriers for the no-bra movement, especially in formal settings where norms are slow to change. Some argue that liberating these norms in professional environments could enhance creative freedom and foster more inclusive workplaces. In this context, the no-bra trend is not merely about personal comfort but also represents a broader challenge to redefine professional and social boundaries—encouraging spaces where all individuals feel they belong, without having to conform to outdated standards.

Navigating these complex social landscapes, the no-bra movement has undeniably catalyzed a dialogue that stretches far beyond personal comfort. It challenges systemic ideas and projects a vision of a future where choices about one's body are respected, free from judgment, and rooted in self-empowerment. As society continues to grapple with the implications of this trend, voices advocating for acceptance and understanding grow louder, urging for progress that reflects empathy, equality, and respect for individuality.

Ultimately, society's reaction to the no-bra trend reflects a broader narrative of change. Change is rarely smooth, often met with resistance, skepticism, and debate. However, it is these very reactions that propel conversations forward, urging society to reflect, question, and, hopefully, evolve. In embracing both the discourse and discomfort that come with it, there emerges an opportunity to reshape societal norms, bringing us closer to a world where women's autonomy over their bodies is not just imagined but realized. As these changes unfold, the no-bra movement stands as a testament to the transformative power of challenging the status quo, spearheading an era where comfort and choice are rightfully prioritized.

Gender and Comfort

Throughout history, societal norms have molded our understanding of gender roles, often conflating femininity with certain expectations and stereotypes. The no-bra movement challenges these established norms, especially as it highlights the interplay between gender and comfort. This trend is not merely about leaving bras behind; it's about redefining how women perceive their own bodies and comfort levels, free from externally imposed expectations.

Traditionally, the discussion around bras was laden with gender-specific expectations, linking their usage to modesty and shaped femininity. However, for many, the bra represents discomfort—a garment that can constrict, irritate, and, paradoxically, detract from a natural appearance. The movement towards not wearing a bra is as much about physical liberation as it is about challenging the societal gaze that dictates female presentation. This shift is a crucial aspect of what many women today term as "body autonomy." It's an act of reclaiming the narrative around what it means to be comfortable in one's own skin.

For those who choose to forego bras, comfort often means rejecting a cycle of social conditioning where femininity is tied to the underwire and molded cup. Instead, the decision is part of a broader personal and cultural transformation. The resistance to cultural pressures often involves questioning why bras have become symbols of femininity and decorum. As society progresses, there's an increasing recognition that comfort should be gender-neutral, allowing each individual to define what comfort means for them without the constraints of traditional gender roles.

The act of choosing comfort over societal norms can feel revolutionary. It compels a reassessment of deeply entrenched ideals, such as why certain garments are perceived as professional or appropriate. Many advocates of the no-bra movement argue that comfort is a fundamental right, not a luxury to be afforded only under certain circumstances. This advocacy extends to workplace attire, demanding spaces that are inclusive and considerate of individual comfort choices.

The movement also catalyzes a significant conversation about how comfort intersects with identity. Gender identity and expression are nuanced, and for many, the choice to abandon traditional garments like bras is part of discovering or honoring their true self. It's a declaration that gender does not have to prescribe discomfort. This perspective has broadened discussions, inviting more inclusive conversations about who gets to define comfort and why.

Amidst these shifts, there's been an influx of media voices and public figures endorsing this narrative, emphasizing personal stories and experiences. These accounts are powerful, often highlighting how choosing comfort has improved quality of life, boosted confidence, and strengthened personal identity. By stepping into the public eye and sharing their stories, these individuals inspire others to reconsider the dictations of gender-specific comfort.

The social implications of rejecting bras are profound, challenging long-standing conventions about gender presentation. By prioritizing comfort, individuals are rejecting the notion that discomfort is an inevitable aspect of femininity. This forms an integral part of wider discussions about body positivity and self-acceptance, urging society to embrace diversity in bodily presentation and comfort preferences.

In navigating the no-bra trend, it's vital to recognize the intersectionality of this movement. For marginalized groups, including those in non-Western cultures, the conversation about comfort and gender can be more complex. These intersections bring to light the diverse ways cultures approach comfort, ultimately contributing to a richer, more nuanced understanding of global comfort norms.

Acknowledging these varying perspectives ensures a dialogue that is inclusive, considering the experiences of those who may not fit neatly into traditional gender binaries or who face different societal pressures. This inclusivity paves the way for a more equitable conversation about what it means to pursue gender and comfort in tandem, freeing individuals from historical constraints and allowing for a more authentic self-expression.

The no-bra movement continues to move the needle on how society perceives gender-related comfort. In championing this cause, individuals are spearheading a shift that could extend beyond bras themselves, ultimately challenging broader gender norms and reconsidering previously unchallenged social scripts. As this trend continues to resonate, it promotes a dynamic discourse about gender and comfort, encouraging society to redefine and expand its understanding of personal freedom and authenticity.

Ultimately, the conversation about gender and comfort is more than about garments—it's about reshaping perceptions and allowing each individual the autonomy to decide what feels right for them. It's an encouragement for society to evolve with its constituents, nurturing spaces that empower choice and celebrate diversity. Such spaces further the dialogue, recognizing the power of gender identity and personal comfort, and creating a world that welcomes all forms of self-expression.

Chapter 5:
Women's Rights and Body Positivity

The journey toward embracing women's rights and body positivity is more than a movement; it's a reclamation of autonomy and dignity. Women's bodies have long been subjected to societal scrutiny and restrictive norms, yet today, we are witnessing a resurgence of empowerment where natural shapes are celebrated rather than suppressed. This chapter delves into the vibrant intersection of women's rights and body positivity, emphasizing how the movement challenges conventional beauty standards and advocates for self-acceptance. By promoting comfort and individual choice, this wave of change empowers women to redefine beauty on their own terms, stripping away the constraints of patriarchal expectations. It's a call to reject judgment and inspire confidence, reminding us that the freedom to choose how we present ourselves is a fundamental right deeply intertwined with broader women's rights issues. In doing so, this chapter aims to illuminate the road to personal freedom and societal change, encouraging a culture that respects and uplifts each woman's unique identity.

Embracing Natural Shapes

The journey towards embracing natural shapes is not just a personal choice but a profound statement in the ongoing conversation about women's rights and body positivity. For centuries, women have been conditioned to view their bodies through a lens of conformity. Society has long dictated the so-called ideal body type, urging women to shape and confine themselves into it. However, the movement to embrace natural shapes challenges these outdated norms and celebrates the diversity of the female body in all its unique forms.

At its core, embracing natural shapes means rejecting the notion that there is a singular, ideal body type. It recognizes that beauty is not linear, nor is it uniform. This mindset fosters a sense of freedom, allowing women to appreciate and accept their bodies as they are, free from societal pressures to alter their natural form. It's about shifting the focus from what the body looks like to what it feels like, emphasizing comfort and health over aesthetics.

Traditionally, bras and other articles of clothing have been used to mold and sculpt women's bodies into shapes deemed desirable by society. They're tools of compliance, often causing physical discomfort and psychological distress. But as women increasingly opt to forgo bras, they're also discarding the societal shackles that bound them. This act of defiance is a step toward body autonomy and a rejection of the patriarchal narratives around femininity and beauty.

Moreover, embracing natural shapes intersects with the broader fight for women's rights. When women embrace their natural forms, they're exerting control over their bodies. It's a declaration of ownership, asserting that their bodies are theirs to adorn, enhance, or embellish as they see fit. This autonomy is a fundamental aspect of women's rights, directly challenging any external attempt to impose standards onto their personal choices.

Inspiration for embracing natural shapes can be found across different cultures and communities. Throughout history, societies have celebrated a plethora of body types, with different regions valuing unique attributes as symbols of beauty and strength. By looking to diverse cultural traditions, women today can find a wealth of alternative narratives that break free from the limitations of mainstream beauty standards.

The No-Bra Movement plays a significant role in the broader acceptance of natural shapes. At its heart, this movement is about the liberation from discomfort and conformity. By choosing to go braless, many women report feeling a sense of freedom and relief, both physically and emotionally. The absence of a bra also becomes a visual and public affirmation of one's acceptance of their natural shape, further fueling the movement's growth and acceptance.

Additionally, embracing natural shapes encourages a more body-positive culture where diversity is appreciated. This cultural shift supports individuals of all sizes and shapes by fostering environments where people feel valued for their authentic selves. It pushes back against industries and media narratives that often perpetuate unrealistic beauty ideals, helping create a space where health and comfort are prioritized over mere appearance.

As more women embrace their natural forms, the impact ripples through various aspects of society. In fashion, for instance, designers are increasingly challenged to create garments that celebrate the natural body rather than reshape it. In workplaces, policies are slowly adapting to recognize and support body positivity, acknowledging that comfort and personal autonomy can lead to more effective and empowered employees.

However, the journey is not without its obstacles. There is still significant resistance from certain quarters that cling to traditional norms. Women who choose to display their natural shape can face criticism or backlash, often rooted in deeply ingrained societal biases. Yet, these challenges further highlight the necessity of this movement and remind us of the powerful role advocacy plays in achieving cultural change.

Embracing natural shapes is a courageous act of self-acceptance, an embodiment of the feminist principle that all women have the right to define and embrace their own bodies on their own terms. It's about understanding that true empowerment comes from within, and it's reflected in how we perceive ourselves and how we treat others.

As women continue to push boundaries and embrace their natural bodies, they inspire others to do the same, cultivating a community of acceptance and empowerment. The call to embrace natural shapes not only celebrates diversity and personal freedom but also paves the way for future generations to live in a world where all forms of femininity are honored and uplifted. In every curve and contour lies a story of reclamation and strength, writing a new chapter in the ongoing dialogue about women's rights and body positivity.

The Intersection with Women's Rights

There's a transformative power in understanding the connection between women's rights and the body positivity movement, especially as it relates to the No-Bra movement. It's a modern surge of empowerment rooted in a long history of struggle for autonomy and equality. Women, for centuries, have faced societal pressures that dictate how they should look, behave, and feel about their bodies. The intersection of these rights and body positivity finds its foundation in challenging these ingrained expectations and advocating for personal choice and freedom.

Body positivity emerged as a response to narrow and often damaging beauty standards. It calls for acceptance of all body types, emphasizing the idea that every body is worthy of love and respect. Within this framework, rejecting the bra symbolizes more than simply opting for comfort. It's about resistance to a patriarchal system that determines a woman's worth based on her appearance. The decision to forego a bra becomes an act of defiance, a statement of self-ownership, and an expression of liberation.

The empowerment derived from these choices ties deeply into broader women's rights issues. Over the years, feminists have worked tirelessly to secure fundamental rights for women, from voting and workplace equality to reproductive rights. Engaging in the No-Bra movement can be seen as a continuation of this fight—a push against oppressive structures and a call for autonomy over one's body. It's about claiming space and voice in a world that has historically sidelined women.

The No-Bra movement does not advocate for the abolition of bras or deem them intrinsically oppressive; rather, it promotes the idea that wearing a bra should be a personal choice, free from judgment and constraint. Likewise, women should have the authority to decide what's best for their body, whether that aligns with societal traditions or not. This acknowledgment of women's agency emphasizes the core of body positivity: empowerment through choice.

Furthermore, the movement highlights important discussions on body shaming and self-esteem. Societal norms often lead to judgment when women choose to go without bras, exposing a double standard related to gender and body image. These judgments are rooted in a culture that idolizes and simultaneously polices the female form. By challenging these perceptions, the No-Bra movement advocates for the dismantling of harmful stereotypes that contend women must conform to specific ideals to be accepted or respected.

Another vital aspect of this intersection is its emphasis on inclusivity. The No-Bra movement recognizes and supports differences in body shapes, sizes, and needs. By accommodating diverse experiences and acknowledging that women may have different reasons for choosing to wear or not wear bras, the movement shines a light on the importance of personal narratives in broader social debates. It encourages a supportive and non-judgmental community, breaking down barriers created by traditional beauty standards.

Equally crucial is the psychological liberation that accompanies these choices. Women's psychological well-being has often been tied to societal acceptance, which demands conformity to certain norms, including wearing bras. By rejecting these pressures, women can reclaim narratives about their bodies, fostering enhanced self-confidence and mental health. Naturally, this shift can lead to improved quality of life, allowing women to prioritize comfort and authenticity over apprehension and judgment.

In workplaces, the fight for bodily autonomy intersects significantly with gender equality. Despite the progress made around gender issues, women still face workplace dress codes rooted in antiquated traditions. Challenging these norms and advocating for clothing choices that prioritize comfort is another dimension of the intersection with women's rights. It pushes for environments where women aren't bound by outdated requirements and can perform with freedom uninfluenced by clothing discomfort.

This intersection also bears significance in legislative changes, as women around the globe, driven by movements like this, demand equality in all facets of life. From changing corporate policies around work attire to advocating for legal rights that protect bodily autonomy, these efforts pave the way for a fairer, more inclusive world. At this crux, personal and political spheres collide, emphasizing how deeply personal choices can drive societal transformation.

Advocacy plays a critical role in driving these conversations. Influential figures and everyday women alike contribute by sharing personal experiences and supporting those on similar journeys. This advocacy underscores a united stand against societal pressures and reinforces the need for solidarity in these issues. Women's rights and body positivity, therefore, are interwoven in a shared battle for recognition, respect, and inclusivity.

Finally, in understanding this intersection, it becomes clear that personal comfort extends far beyond individual declinations of norms. It's a collective step towards equality, where women's rights are not compartmentalized as distinct from social or personal well-being. The intersection with women's rights redefines success as personal happiness and autonomy, aligning the No-Bra movement with the broader goals of feminist struggles.

Chapter 6:
Stories from the No-Bra Movement

Embedded within the fabric of the no-bra movement are compelling stories that weave together diverse experiences and influential voices. Women from various backgrounds have shared narratives of liberation, challenging the longstanding dictates of fashion and societal expectations. Take, for instance, the account of one young professional who discovered a newfound sense of self-assuredness by foregoing bras. Her story is echoed by countless others who found empowerment by embracing comfort over conformity. Influencers and pioneers of the movement have amplified these voices, highlighting the deeply personal reasons behind this shift. These stories are not just anecdotes; they are powerful testaments to the movement's impact, illustrating how personal choices can ripple through cultures and redefine norms. Each narrative is a beacon for those still tethered to outdated standards, lighting a path toward a more authentic state of being, one that honors both comfort and agency.

Personal Experiences

Every woman who's chosen to embrace the no-bra movement has a unique story to tell—stories that intertwine personal revelation and societal challenge. Many begin their journeys quietly, often as a personal quest for comfort that gradually transforms into a bold statement. These experiences underscore a universal theme: the pursuit of personal comfort can be both an internal revolution and a powerful social act.

Take the experience of Emma, a young professional in a bustling city. Working long hours in a high-pressure environment, she often felt restricted—physically and metaphorically—under her tailored suits and structured bras. The decision to ditch the bra wasn't immediate, nor was it easy. She worried about judgment from coworkers, fearing whispers about her professionalism. Yet, after a particularly grueling day, comfort won out over convention. Despite her apprehension, she spent the next day at work feeling liberated. The absence of underwire felt like the lifting of a heavy shroud. What surprised Emma the most wasn't just the comfort but the confidence. She walked taller, her shoulders squared with a newfound sense of self-acceptance.

Emma realized that her comfort didn't diminish her professionalism; rather, it enhanced her presence. She shared, "I felt like me, perhaps for the first time in my career. And that authenticity, it spilled into my work." Her story reflects a broader realization that comfort can coexist with competence, challenging traditional notions of workplace etiquette.

Similarly, Anaya, a mother of two from the suburbs, found the conventional bra increasingly burdensome after her pregnancies. She initially struggled with societal standards of femininity and nurture, feeling caught between them. Each morning, she wrestled with the inner conflict of conforming to the status quo versus pursuing personal ease, a battle that many women can relate to—especially in the postpartum phase where body image concerns often peak.

Her turning point came unexpectedly, during a calm afternoon at home, observing her children play. As they dashed around carelessly, unburdened by the world's expectations, Anaya realized she deserved that same freedom from constraint. She stopped wearing bras entirely, embracing her natural form. What she discovered was an enhancement of her maternal instincts—not a weakening. "Being comfortable in my own skin," she observed, "allowed me to be more present with my kids." Her bold choice ignited conversations among her peers, many of whom had silently echoed her struggles.

Not all experiences stem from professional or maternal pressures. For some, like Jess, a college student balancing the weights of academia and social life, going braless was an unexpected venture into self-discovery. She stumbled upon the concept through social media, where influential voices challenged body norms. Intrigued, Jess cautiously decided to experiment. During this transitional phase of life, where students often redefine their identities, she found herself questioning long-held beliefs about beauty and propriety.

Initially, Jess applied the no-bra decision sporadically. At parties, where dress codes were looser, she tested the waters, finding comfort with every trial. When a friend complimented her for seeming so at ease on a night out, Jess realized this simple act empowered her social persona. It was as if unveiling her natural self revealed layers of authenticity that resonated deeply with those around her. "The confidence was addictive," Jess reflected. "It transformed into a kind of armor, not one that concealed, but one that made me proud of who I am."

Then there's Sarah, who dealt with medical reasons for her choice. After undergoing breast surgery, she found the typical structure of bras intolerable. Facing a non-negotiable circumstance, Sarah initially lamented her loss of choice. Yet, over time, she learned to embrace her body's needs, letting her physical comfort guide her rather than societal rules. Her journey is a poignant reminder of the complex relationship many women have with bras—a symbol of health, beauty, and sometimes, restriction.

Healing, both physically and psychologically, Sarah shared, "I realized I wasn't opting out of something. I was choosing to take care of myself." Her story highlights the importance of kindness to one's body, an approach sometimes forgotten in the race to meet societal expectations.

These personal experiences showcase an array of motivations and outcomes, yet they converge on a singular truth: the journey to comfort is deeply personal and inherently empowering. Each woman's narrative is a testament to the courage it takes to challenge ingrained norms and embrace one's authentic self. The movement is as much about individual empowerment as it is about collective solidarity. It invites women everywhere to redefine beauty and comfort—one unhooked bralette at a time.

The courageous steps of Emma, Anaya, Jess, and Sarah inspire those around them to question, to wonder, and importantly, to act. These women exemplify a quiet revolution, one that reverberates loudly in challenging societal norms and celebrating body autonomy. Their voices, once hesitant, now resonate with power and a shared commitment to living truthfully. Their stories are living proof that comfort isn't just a personal preference; it's a personal right.

Ultimately, these narratives of personal defiance and acceptance forge paths for future generations. They craft a legacy—one quilted with tales of freedom, truth, and above all, the courage to be comfortable in one's own skin. They show that the no-bra movement isn't merely a reaction; it's a profound declaration of self-worth and dignity.

Influential Voices

The No-Bra Movement is not just a fleeting trend or a societal quirk. It's a powerful moment in the ongoing dialogue about women's rights, body autonomy, and cultural conceptions of comfort. At its core, this movement stands on the shoulders of those influential voices who dared to speak up and inspire others. Some women took the mic, some shared their stories in intimate circles, and others used the power of the pen. These trailblazers have each left an indelible mark on the movement, breaking barriers and challenging the status quo.

In the early days, long before hashtags and online communities, personal conviction often pushed voices to the forefront. Consider the pioneers of the women's liberation movement who, in the 1960s and 1970s, questioned every aspect of societal conformity. It wasn't just about defiance; it was a pursuit of personal freedom and comfort. These women laid the groundwork, planting seeds of thought that would bloom into today's no-bra discussions.

One cannot overlook the cultural critics who brought attention to the rigidity of gender norms. Their critiques offered a lens through which to view the bra not merely as a garment of support, but as a symbol of imposed femininity. They highlighted how societal expectations often disconnected women from their bodily autonomy, making it less about choice and more about compliance. Such voices articulated a powerful narrative: comfort should never be forsaken in the name of so-called propriety.

Then there are the storytellers, those who wove personal narratives that resonated deeply with countless women worldwide. These stories are marked by vulnerability and authenticity—women who shared their initial insecurities about stepping out sans bra, and subsequently, their newfound confidence and comfort. Sharing tales of liberation, they encouraged solidarity. After all, when one woman found comfort, it created a ripple effect, emboldening others to explore their own comfort zones.

Intersectionality has been a critical component, too. Influential voices from marginalized communities brought inclusive perspectives, reminding everyone that the movement isn't monolithic. They pose essential questions: How does race alter the perception of going braless? In what ways do cultural backgrounds influence understandings of modesty? These voices challenge the notion that the no-bra movement is a uniform experience, urging a deeper examination of how various identities intersect in the pursuit of comfort.

Let's consider the thought leaders and academics who scrutinized the very fabric of societal norms. By leveraging research and data, they provided compelling evidence linking body autonomy with psychological well-being. Their studies amplified the narrative that bras, once deemed necessary, might not be as crucial as once thought. This scholarly backing lends confidence to the voices advocating for personal choice and emphasizes that comfort isn't trivial—it's a legitimate aspect of women's health.

Furthermore, those voices with platforms—celebrities, influencers, and social media mavens—have undeniably played a significant role in popularizing the movement. When well-known figures choose to embrace a braless lifestyle, audiences take note. It ignites conversations, both supportive and critical, propelling the movement into broader cultural consciousness. However, it's crucial to recognize that with visibility comes responsibility. These influential figures must navigate their platforms thoughtfully, ensuring they respect the diverse experiences within the movement.

The movement also celebrates corpo-activists —those within the fashion industry who proposed bras that prioritize comfort or offered alternative styles that challenge traditional bra designs. By recognizing the market's capacity for choice, these voices provided tangible options, transforming abstract ideals into practical realities. They've shown that comfort and style needn't be mutually exclusive, encouraging a shift in how undergarments are perceived and consumed.

We cannot disregard the voices of dissent, which, in many ways, fortify the movement. Critics challenge the no-bra ethos, arguing from perspectives of modesty, tradition, or perceived necessity. It's these voices that push advocates to refine their arguments, ensuring the movement's foundations are robust and inclusive. Engaging with opposition often solidifies the movement's objectives and strengthens its resolve.

For many, the realization that going bra-free is akin to an act of rebellion against oppressive norms is empowering. This isn't simply a rejection of a piece of clothing—it's about reclaiming power over one's own body. The influential voices of the movement constantly echo this sentiment, giving strength to those who listen. Their stories are a testament to the profound impact one individual's decision can have on both personal well-being and broader societal change.

Finally, the enduring effect of these voices lies in their ability to inspire. They serve as a call to action; a reminder that each person's comfort journey is unique yet interwoven into a collective pursuit of autonomy. By highlighting these narratives, they invite more voices to join the conversation, fostering a community that champions choice and celebrates diversity in comfort over conformity.

As the movement evolves, new voices will undoubtedly rise with fresh perspectives and experiences. What remains steadfast is the undying commitment to advancing the discourse on comfort, autonomy, and the right to choose. The influential voices of today assure us that the conversation is alive and well, continually reshaping how we embrace bodies, choices, and freedom.

Chapter 7:
Fashion and the No-Bra Trend

The intersection of fashion and the no-bra trend marks a significant shift in how society views women's comfort and self-expression. Breaking free from traditional style constraints, this movement embraces natural silhouettes and challenges designers to reconsider their approach to women's apparel. As high fashion and everyday wear alike begin to celebrate body autonomy, the trend redefines what it means to be stylish and empowered. Designers now tantalizingly explore innovative materials and structures that not only flatter the female form but also prioritize comfort. The ripple effect is causing a reevaluation of current style standards, urging the fashion industry to focus on inclusivity and authenticity over conformity. This collective move towards embracing personal freedom signals a pivotal transformation in the way women dress and perceive their bodies, reinforcing that true beauty stems from confidence and self-acceptance.

Changing Style Standards

The fashion world, with its ever-shifting trends and norms, has long been a dynamic field that both reflects and influences cultural attitudes. As we step into the realm of changing style standards, particularly regarding the no-bra trend, it's essential to understand how these shifts mark a significant departure from past conventions. This evolution in fashion is more than just a change in clothing choices; it's a statement, an assertion of identity, and a defiance against traditional expectations.

For years, the bra has been seen as a staple of modern women's attire, representing both support and a societal standard of femininity. However, as cultural dialogues evolve, so too do the expectations surrounding what women choose to wear. The no-bra movement— part of a broader push for autonomy and body acceptance—challenges the sartorial status quo that has dominated for decades.

The emergence of the no-bra trend aligns with an overarching shift toward comfort-driven fashion. Historically, women's clothing has often favored form over function, placing aesthetics above comfort. This paradigm is now being questioned. Women are choosing garments that prioritize their personal comfort without sacrificing style. In this context, the decision to forgo a bra is as much about rejecting discomfort as it is about embracing one's natural shape.

In recent years, designers and brands have responded to these shifting preferences by offering more inclusive clothing lines—styles that cater to a diversity of body types and personal choices. We're seeing an increasing number of fashion houses that understand the importance of versatility and comfort in their designs. This shift isn't just about producing bra-free options; it's about creating entire collections that celebrate the myriad ways women express their individuality.

The no-bra trend also brings to light the broader discussion of fashion's role in societal constructs of beauty. For decades, advertising and media have perpetuated a narrow definition of beauty, one often characterized by rigid standards. The movement towards embracing comfort and self-expression offers a counter-narrative, one where beauty is multifaceted, and where each individual's choice is celebrated rather than scrutinized.

Moreover, the change in style standards has encouraged a dialogue on sustainability within the fashion industry. Fast fashion's relentless demand often prioritizes quantity over quality, contributing to environmental concerns. As more individuals and designers advocate for conscious fashion choices, the emphasis shifts toward sustainable practices, including the creation of durable, comfortable clothing that lessens environmental impact.

This revolution in style also intersects with broader social movements advocating for gender equality and women's rights. As women demand the right to make choices based on their comfort and preference, they're simultaneously challenging the archaic norms that have policed their bodies and attire. The no-bra trend thus becomes a symbol of empowerment, encouraging women to listen to their bodies and make choices that align with their own comfort, not societal expectations.

It's important to understand that changing style standards go beyond just clothing. They embody a shift towards inclusivity, where diverse experiences and voices are acknowledged and valued in fashion narratives. This movement calls into question the very foundation of fashion norms, asking us to consider who sets these standards and why we've adhered to them for so long.

The no-bra movement doesn't solely aim to discard bras entirely or to demonize them but rather to provide options—allowing every individual to make choices that best suit their own body and lifestyle. For some, bras will continue to be a source of comfort and support, while for others, abandoning them will be liberating. The focus is on choice, respect, and individuality.

As we contemplate the future of fashion, it's clear that evolving style standards are part of a larger cultural revolution, one where comfort, sustainability, and personal autonomy are at the forefront. The conversation about bras and style continues, shaping not only the garments we wear but also the society we inhabit. In embracing changing style standards, we're not just choosing new fabrics and cuts; we're choosing a new narrative, one that empowers and uplifts women everywhere.

Designer Perspectives

In the ever-evolving world of fashion, designers hold a unique position. They're the visionaries shaping not just clothing but the collective cultural dialogue surrounding body image and autonomy. With the no-bra trend gaining momentum, these industry leaders are embracing this movement, forging new paths that celebrate comfort and authenticity. Their perspectives reveal a radical shift from structured expectation to intentional liberation.

At the heart of this shift is the idea of clothing that honors the natural form. Many designers are moving away from rigid, constrictive garments towards styles that allow freedom of movement and expression. This transition isn't just about removing a bra; it's a holistic approach to fashion that prioritizes how women feel in their clothes over how they look. It's a powerful statement in an industry historically characterized by dictating rather than liberating.

Some designers argue that the no-bra trend is more than a fashion statement—it's a social manifesto. For leaders in the fashion industry, acknowledging the no-bra movement means tapping into broader social changes. These designers are redefining aesthetics to include softness and strength, autonomy, and authenticity. They recognize the beauty in diversity and the empowerment that comes with a self-directed wardrobe. As a result, collections are beginning to feature a range of silhouettes that don't presume to standardize or restrain.

With comfort as their muse, designers are experimenting with new materials and technologies. Fabrics that breathe and stretch, tailored construction without tight seams or wires, and innovative layering techniques are paving the way for this trend to thrive. This experimentation extends into the realm of bespoke tailoring, where designers create personalized experiences that accommodate diverse body shapes and preferences without reverting to traditional structures.

Fashion shows and catalogs are now telling a different story. Gone are the days when runways demanded uniformity in presentation. Instead, designers are sending models down the runway who exude individuality and confidence, whether they choose to wear bras or not. This choice serves as a statement that comfort is not a compromise on style; on the contrary, it enhances it. These visual narratives are powerful, showing that fashion can embrace comfort as a core value, and contribute to changing attitudes worldwide.

Renowned designer Claire T. has been vocal about her inspiration from ancient dress styles that prioritize ease and form over fashion rigidity. She emphasizes how these historical designs offer valuable lessons, proving that comfort and aesthetics have always been intertwined. Other designers find inspiration in the natural movements of the body, adapting their creations to work with, rather than against, its contours.

Some critics argue that the no-bra trend won't last, seeing it as a fleeting fad more than an enduring transformation. However, designers advocating for it believe otherwise, pointing to its deep roots in changing societal norms about women's rights and freedoms. For them, this isn't just about garments; it's about changing perceptions and promoting healthier relationships with one's body.

Designers are increasingly using their platforms to engage directly with consumers, inviting feedback and fostering conversations about what women truly want and need from their clothing. This interaction not only informs their creative process but also empowers consumers by validating their preferences and experiences. They believe fashion should not just follow trends but foster them, creating environments where comfort and individuality are celebrated.

In terms of economic impact, embracing the no-bra trend can be seen as a savvy move. As consumer demand shifts towards comfortable, sustainable apparel, designers aligned with these values are poised to benefit. This doesn't only apply to high fashion; everyday wear brands are also responding by creating options that speak to a new, comfort-first shopping mindset.

The industry's support of the no-bra trend highlights a growing commitment to inclusivity. Designers are increasingly using their influence to break down traditional fashion barriers, offering options that cater to a wider range of needs and desires. They understand that supporting comfort goes beyond the physical—it is about making statements about equality, respect, and personhood.

For a designer like Julian M., celebrating imperfection is key. His collections focus on the idea that each piece of clothing can tell a story, reflecting the unique lives and experiences of those who wear them. By doing so, Julian hopes to inspire a shift in perspective where fashion becomes a medium for self-discovery and expression, not merely adherence to status quo.

As the dialogue evolves, the consensus among many designers is that the integration of the no-bra trend into mainstream fashion symbolizes a broader, fundamental change. This movement not only addresses physical comfort but challenges entrenched norms, encouraging women to reclaim their bodies and choices. The works of these designers encapsulate an industry at the forefront of transformation, inviting all to embrace a more liberated form of expression.

Chapter 8:
The Role of Media and Advertising

In the intricate dance between societal norms and emerging movements, media and advertising have always held the spotlight, shaping perceptions and fostering change, often in subtle yet profound ways. When it comes to the No-Bra movement, these forces play a pivotal role, balancing traditional beauty standards with burgeoning calls for authenticity and body autonomy. Media outlets have the power to redefine what is considered acceptable and beautiful, often mirroring or challenging the status quo. Advertising, with its pervasive reach, can either reinforce outdated stereotypes or champion diverse, empowering narratives that challenge the binding expectations placed on women. Although the journey towards widespread acceptance of the movement involves untangling years of ingrained biases and commercial agendas, the shifts in media representations hint at a promising future where female comfort and natural form are celebrated rather than constrained.

Media Representation

Media representation plays a pivotal role in shaping public perceptions and attitudes towards societal movements, including the no-bra movement. It's no secret that the world's view of women and femininity has been and continues to be largely influenced by the media. Over the years, media outlets have wielded immense power, often dictating what is considered acceptable, beautiful, or even normal. In doing so, they've also contributed to the stigmatization or normalization of various body image standards and clothing choices.

The roots of current media portrayals can be traced back to traditional advertising campaigns, which often reinforced stereotypical images of femininity. Women were typically depicted in ways that prioritized physical aesthetics over comfort, subtly (and sometimes not so subtly) suggesting that adhering to these ideals was paramount. This ingrained notion—appearing a certain way for public approval—has fueled the lingerie industry for decades, with bras marketed as essential to achieving the societal standard of beauty.

However, the recent rise of the no-bra movement highlights how media representation can evolve, showcasing a shift in focus from appearance to comfort and empowerment. Social media platforms, in particular, have become arenas where women can share their stories, offering a counter-narrative to mainstream media's traditionally narrow views. These platforms provide a space for voices that advocate for body positivity and autonomy, challenging longstanding norms.

Despite this shift, the portrayal of the no-bra movement in mainstream media remains complex. On one hand, there are narratives that celebrate personal choice and self-expression, casting the decision to forgo bras in a positive, liberating light. On the other hand, some media outlets continue to sensationalize or trivialize the movement, reducing it to a mere fashion statement or attention-seeking behavior rather than a legitimate expression of bodily autonomy.

Advertising also plays a crucial role in media representation. Brands are increasingly aligning themselves with messages of empowerment and body positivity to appeal to a more conscious consumer base. This trend has resulted in some advertising campaigns spotlighting women who choose comfort over conformity. Such campaigns can offer powerful endorsements for the no-bra movement, influencing public perception by presenting diversity in forms, shapes, and preferences as not just acceptable but commendable.

Notably, the impact of advertising goes beyond simply selling a product. It also mirrors and molds cultural attitudes, shaping how society views issues of gender, freedom of choice, and self-expression. Advertisements that captivate with authenticity and inclusivity can drive the narrative towards a more open-minded acceptance of diverse comfort and fashion choices. However, the risk of commodification is ever-present. When movements are used purely as marketing strategies without genuine commitment to the underlying causes, there is the danger of reducing significant issues to trends that lose their essence.

Television shows and movies are also major players in media representation, portraying scenarios that may either reinforce or challenge societal norms regarding women's bodies and clothing choices. When characters in popular media are depicted embracing a bra-free lifestyle, it subtly endorses the choice as normal. Such depictions can not only influence public attitudes but also legitimize the movement in the eyes of viewers, many of whom look to media for cues on acceptable behavior.

Yet, it's essential to recognize that these portrayals are uneven. While some works offer progressive narratives, others still fall into the trap of exploiting femininity for entertainment, focusing excessively on physical appearance and policing women's choices. How media chooses to present or ignore the no-bra movement and similar advocacies reveals much about ongoing power dynamics in cultural dialogue.

The media is a powerful tool for storytelling, capable of bringing to light the nuances of the no-bra movement. It's crucial that this power is wielded mindfully, amplifying diverse voices and acknowledging the multifaceted reasons women might choose to eschew traditional bra-wearing norms. Through informed representation, media can transcend stereotypes, fostering a cultural environment that respects individuality and personal comfort.

Ultimately, media representation of the no-bra movement can be both liberating and limiting. As readers become more critical consumers of media, they hold the capacity to influence future portrayals. By supporting and demanding narratives that are rooted in truth and represent genuine empowerment, society can push media producers towards more responsible and inclusive storytelling, leading to a broader acceptance of diverse expressions of comfort and body autonomy.

Impact of Advertising

In a world saturated with images and messages, advertising wields an immense influence on our perceptions of beauty, comfort, and empowerment. This is especially true when it comes to societal norms and expectations surrounding women's bodies. Advertising has long played a dual role in shaping and reflecting cultural attitudes, often perpetuating stereotypes while also potentially challenging them. Its impact on the No-Bra movement is as complex as it is significant.

Historically, advertising has reinforced the idea that women's bodies need to be controlled and molded to fit narrow definitions of acceptability. Bra advertisements, for instance, have traditionally presented bras as essential for femininity, elegance, and even moral decency. These ads often project the image that wearing a bra aligns with being put-together and respectable, subtly suggesting that a woman's worth is tied to her adherence to these norms. In doing so, they cemented the bra as an unquestioned staple in women's wardrobes.

Despite these rigid portrayals, advertising also possesses the inherent power to drive change. As societal perspectives shift, so too can the messages that are sent through media. In recent years, there has been a noticeable transformation in advertising strategies, prompted by a growing demand for authenticity and inclusivity. Brands are increasingly embracing messages of body positivity, self-acceptance, and empowerment. Their campaigns frequently feature diverse body types and advocate for comfort over conformity, challenging the long-held belief that bras are a necessary component of womanhood.

One of the most profound impacts of advertising on the No-Bra movement is its ability to reach a vast and varied audience. By publicly acknowledging and representing the choice not to wear a bra, advertisers can normalize this decision and encourage discussions about why women might opt for comfort and autonomy over traditional expectations. This visibility can empower individuals to make choices that are true to themselves, rather than feeling constrained by outdated norms.

However, not all advertising is created equal, and there's a critical distinction between genuine advocacy and surface-level marketing. Some brands might co-opt body positivity and empowerment themes without truly committing to the values they claim to support. It's important for consumers to be discerning and to support companies that demonstrate a genuine commitment to these principles beyond their marketing efforts.

Moreover, advertising's impact isn't solely in its ability to sell products; it's also in its narrative-shaping power. When advertisements reinforce that comfort and autonomy are acceptable choices, they challenge the societal script that women have been conditioned to follow. These messages can have a liberating effect, reducing the stigma around choosing not to wear a bra and validating personal comfort as a legitimate preference.

The rise of social media has added another layer to this dynamic, amplifying diverse voices and perspectives that may have previously been marginalized in traditional advertising spaces. Platforms like

Instagram and Twitter allow individuals to share their personal stories and experiences with the No-Bra movement, creating organic advertising that often resonates more deeply with audiences. This democratization of media can help dismantle the traditional power structures of advertising, placing narrative control back into the hands of individuals.

At its core, the evolution of advertising in relation to the No-Bra movement reflects broader societal changes. As more women reject the notion that their bodies should be policed by others, advertising adapts and evolves. This transformation isn't merely a response to market demands; it signals a profound cultural shift towards body autonomy and empowerment. Advertisers that successfully harness this spirit do more than promote a product—they facilitate a movement that respects and celebrates individuality and comfort.

Nonetheless, there remains a tension between advertising's commercial objectives and its capacity for social influence. Ads still primarily serve the goal of selling products, and the sincerity of their messages can sometimes come into question. This underscores the importance of consumer awareness and critical engagement with media messages. When consumers hold advertisers accountable, demanding authenticity and genuine advocacy, change becomes not just possible but probable.

In conclusion, while advertising has historically played a role in upholding restrictive norms about women's bodies, it also holds the potential to dismantle these narratives. As advertisers continue to embrace more inclusive and empowering messages, they contribute to the normalization of diverse experiences and choices, including the decision to go bra-free. This not only helps validate and uplift individual choices but also challenges the collective cultural consciousness, paving the way for a more inclusive and autonomous understanding of comfort and empowerment.

As we move forward, the relationship between advertising and cultural norms will likely continue to evolve. Advertising's impact on the No-Bra movement is just one example of its intricate role in shaping societal attitudes. By fostering dialogue and embracing diverse narratives, advertising can become a powerful ally in the ongoing quest for body positivity, autonomy, and true empowerment for all women. The journey may be complex, but the potential for meaningful change is undeniable as long as the messages remain authentic and aligned with the evolving values of society.

Chapter 9:
Cultural Attitudes Towards Female Comfort

The journey towards embracing female comfort within cultural contexts is as diverse as it is profound. Across the globe, attitudes towards women's bodily autonomy and comfort have been shaped by historical, social, and economic influences, and they vary widely. In some cultures, the idea of comfort is interwoven with traditional values, while in others, it's seen as a form of rebellion against the status quo. Historically, female comfort often took a backseat, overshadowed by societal norms dictating modesty and decorum. Yet, as the world witnesses a shift from rigid conventions to more inclusive narratives, women are reclaiming their right to comfort, irrespective of long-standing stereotypes. This cultural metamorphosis challenges conventions and encourages a re-evaluation of how comfort is perceived and prioritized. By understanding these diverse cultural attitudes, we can appreciate the nuances of the global comfort conversation, acknowledging that while progress is palpable, unified change requires a commitment to continuing this dialogue across all borders.

Cross-Cultural Comparisons

It's fascinating how cultural perceptions shape women's choices regarding comfort and autonomy, especially when it comes to discarding bras. Across various societies, the no-bra movement presents distinct challenges and differing levels of acceptance. These attitudes are deeply rooted in historical, social, and religious contexts.

In Western countries, where individualism often holds sway, the no-bra movement has gained significant traction. Here, the ideal of personal freedom meshes with feminist ideals, advocating not just for liberation from lingerie but from any societal expectations dictating what women should wear. Celebrities and influencers often lead the charge, challenging conventional beauty standards and encouraging women to prioritize comfort over societal norms. This attitude prevails in many liberal societies where personal expression is valued highly.

Interestingly, while some countries in Asia like Japan and South Korea embrace elements of Western fashion and culture, when it comes to women's attire, traditional views often prevail. Many women still feel pressure to conform to conservative dress codes, influenced by long-standing societal expectations. However, younger generations in urban areas are beginning to challenge these norms, drawing inspiration from global trends and advocating for choice and comfort.

Switching geographical lenses, in sub-Saharan Africa, perspectives on female comfort and attire are as diverse as the cultures themselves. In some communities, societal expectations around modesty can restrict women's choices. Yet, in others, traditional attires that offer comfort and freedom have always been accepted and celebrated. The influence of global movements and access to international media are steadily changing mindsets, creating a unique blend of traditional and contemporary views.

Latin American societies exhibit a complex interplay between traditional values and modern, progressive ideologies. In some parts, the aesthetic appreciation of form-fitting clothing remains prevalent, making the journey towards accepting no-bra choices a challenging path. Yet, as discussions around body positivity and feminism gain momentum, a rise in the acceptance of personal comfort over perceived societal obligations has been observed. Urban centers are particularly vibrant spaces where these discussions flourish and where personal choice is increasingly celebrated.

In many Middle Eastern cultures, historical and religious influences significantly affect dress codes and attitudes towards female comfort. For women here, dressing practices are often tied to cultural or religious identity, and stepping outside these norms can be seen as controversial. However, movements advocating for women's rights and choice are gaining voices even in these regions. It's a nuanced conversation that respects tradition while questioning whether these norms best serve women today.

In Europe, the cultural mosaic sees varying views even within its continental boundaries. Northern European countries, with their progressive social policies and focus on gender equality, generally support women's comfort choices, including opting out of wearing bras. Conversely, Southern Europe showcases a diverse mix of tradition and modernity, where social norms continue to shape fashion and comfort choices in complicated ways.

Australia and New Zealand often align with Western cultural attitudes, promoting individual choice and celebrating diversity in dress as part of a broader discourse on women's rights. This openness encourages women to express themselves freely, challenging norms that don't resonate with their personal values.

In countries like India, the dichotomy between urban and rural perspectives is stark. Urban areas, influenced by Western ideals and the digital revolution, see more women advocating for comfort and body autonomy. Rural regions, however, often adhere to traditional values where women's attire is dictated by conservative societal norms.

From these cultural crossroads, it's evident that attitudes towards female comfort are not just about clothing but are deeply intertwined with broader cultural, historical, and socio-political narratives. As global awareness of the no-bra movement spreads, it interacts with these narratives, sometimes affirming, sometimes challenging them.

What is universal, however, is the underlying pursuit of personal autonomy and comfort. Each society's journey is unique, flavored by its history and values. Yet, the overarching trend points towards a future where women worldwide can make personal comfort choices without fear of judgment. This shift signifies progress not just for women but for societies as a whole, as they reflect on and challenge the norms shaping their worldviews.

Historical Views on Female Comfort

Understanding the historical views on female comfort requires diving into a complex tapestry of cultural, social, and economic factors that have shaped women's lives throughout the ages. The pursuit of comfort, particularly in clothing, has often been tied closely with the prevailing societal norms and expectations of femininity. Historically, women's bodies have been subjected to stringent standards that prioritize aesthetics or societal expectations over comfort and health.

In many ancient civilizations, women's clothing served as a marker of status and adherence to cultural norms. During the Greco-Roman era, women's attire was often designed to emphasize the idealized female form. The tight-fitting and layered garments did not prioritize personal comfort, largely because a woman's appearance was seen as an extension of her family's honor and social standing. Comfort, as it relates to personal clothing, was often a secondary or even tertiary concern.

The Middle Ages brought about the corset, a symbol that persisted over centuries as a testament to how female comfort was sacrificed at the altar of beauty. Corsets were rigid and restrictive, meant to shape the torso into an artifice of societal ideals. Despite the physical discomfort and potential health risks, these garments persisted, highlighting a period where the silhouette—an outward expression endorsed by male-dominated societal standards—was valued more than the wellbeing of women. The corset became an emblematic device of female oppression, demonstrating how comfort was consistently compromised for appearance.

With the dawn of the industrial revolution and the subsequent expansion of the textile industry, women's attire began to subtly shift. The influx of ready-made garments introduced new fabrics and designs, allowing for marginal increases in accessibility to comfortable clothing. Yet, even then, comfort often remained elusive for women, tethered to the backseat as fashion took precedence. The prevailing wisdom echoed that women must adorn themselves in a manner that suited public taste, not personal ease.

The 20th century marked a significant shift, intersecting with broader movements for women's rights and changes in societal roles. During the 1920s, the flapper era introduced looser-fitting clothing, offering women a taste of freedom and comfort. It coincided with a cultural revolution that saw women stepping into domains previously dominated by men, whether in the workplace or social spaces. This loosening of social restrictions also allowed for a defiance of sartorial norms that had strangled comfort for centuries. However, much of this rebellion was momentary as the conservative backlash of the 1950s reintroduced more restrictive clothing styles, albeit without the extreme discomfort of prior eras.

The feminist movements of the 1960s and 1970s revived conversations about female comfort, both physically and socially. These decades challenged the status quo, advocating for authenticity in self-presentation. Women increasingly sought to redefine comfort, not just as a physical state but as a social right. The bra-burning myth, while exaggerative, symbolized a bold rejection of attire that policed women's comfort. It highlighted a growing awareness and demand for clothing that catered to an authentic experience of the female form.

Despite these shifts, the dialogue around female comfort and attire continues to be fraught with challenges. Today's cultural attitudes are reflective of a complex interplay between historical hangovers and modern advancements. The no-bra movement, a contemporary reflection of these evolving views, underscores ongoing debates regarding autonomy, comfort, and societal expectations. It's an act of personal choice that invites reflection on how far society has traveled concerning female comfort and how much further it needs to go.

Historical views on female comfort cannot be disentangled from the broader historical context of women's rights. As the liberated movements of the 21st century take shape, advocating for personal choice becomes intrinsically linked to comfort. This era presents itself as a culmination of past struggles and present-day activism, empowering women to rewrite clothing norms.

While modern society takes comfort for granted, for women, achieving this state has been a hard-fought journey. Through historical narratives, it becomes evident that the path to comfort is part revolution, part evolution—each woman's choice to embrace comfort adding another chapter to this ongoing story. The persistent struggle illustrates that comfort isn't merely changing clothes; it's challenging the very fabric of cultural norms and redefining them holistically, consciously, and continuously.

Chapter 10:
Empowerment and Body Autonomy

Empowerment and body autonomy have become powerful rallying cries in the ongoing redefinition of what it means to embrace one's personal freedom. The no-bra movement highlights a growing awareness among women to claim sovereignty over their own bodies, challenging an age-old societal script that dictates conformity. This modern discourse isn't merely about shedding a piece of clothing; it's a profound movement geared towards liberating women from the societal shackles that have long dictated femininity and comfort. Embodying a spirit of resilience, women are penning personal narratives that align with their authentic selves, creating a space where choice reigns supreme. In cultivating body autonomy, they inspire others to listen to their bodies' unique desires and redefine empowerment on their own terms, illustrating that true freedom comes not from adhering to imposed standards but from owning one's journey unapologetically.

Redefining Empowerment

In today's evolving cultural landscape, empowerment is no longer a distant ideal but a tangible force reshaping how we see ourselves and our bodies. The journey to redefine empowerment is inherently tied to the quest for body autonomy, a principle advocating that women should have the right to make choices about their bodies without external pressures or societal constraints. This chapter, situated within the larger conversation of comfort and self-acceptance, delves into the role of empowerment as a critical axis around which body autonomy revolves.

Empowerment today means embracing a spectrum of personal choices, including the decision to wear or not wear a bra. For many, the simple act of choosing comfort over societal expectations acts as a statement of personal freedom. Women are challenging the preconceived notions embedded in cultural narratives that often equate femininity with constraint, breaking free from the dictates of conventional standards. This act of defiance is not just about discarding undergarments but about reclaiming control over one's own body.

Across generations, empowerment has been wielded as a term that, at times, seemed elusive and broad. However, the modern redefinition aligns it closely with tangible actions like body autonomy. This has inspired a more profound understanding of individual rights, focusing on personal choice as a form of strength. Consider the countless stories of women who have publicly shared their experiences, from defying dress codes to advocating for personal comfort. Their narratives illuminate the path of empowerment, underscoring that it starts with self-awareness and courage.

This redefinition moves beyond a singular focus on gender, embracing a more inclusive understanding of comfort that challenges traditional gender roles. These changing dynamics reflect broader societal shifts, where empowerment serves as an equalizing force, inviting everyone to reimagine comfort free from restrictive norms. Today, the dialogue around empowerment echoes louder, fueled by social movements and feminist discourse that prioritize individual voice and choice above oppressive conventions.

Empowerment, seen through the lens of body autonomy, becomes a personal revolution. It calls for a shift from passive acceptance to active engagement in personal decision-making. For many women, choosing to participate in the No-Bra movement, for instance, is an act of personal liberation from the physical discomfort and societal surveillance tied to prescribed appearances. It represents a move towards living authentically, syncing the outer expression with inner values.

Providing women with the autonomy to define their own standards of beauty and comfort translates into a radical act of self-love and acceptance. This empowerment promotes the message that every body is unique and deserving of respect and acknowledgment—not for what it adorns or conforms to, but for its inherent sovereignty. The movement urges women to listen to their own needs and desires, refuting the homogenized concepts of femininity.

For the movement to gain a foothold and create lasting change, cultural attitudes need to evolve. Here, empowerment is not just about dismantling old structures but constructing new paradigms that prioritize inclusivity and authenticity. Educational campaigns, storytelling, and advocacy play instrumental roles in achieving this goal. Empowerment aligns with education because informed choices bolster the autonomy that underlies it, creating a cycle of continuous growth.

With each passing day, more voices rise in unison, underscoring that true empowerment is woven through the everyday actions we take and the decisions we make for our own well-being. It's about feeling empowered to walk through the world on your terms, unfettered by societal shackles or judgment. Through this lens, not only does empowerment redefine personal autonomy, but it also reshapes collective consciousness, steering the world towards a more inclusive understanding of autonomy and equal rights.

Redefining empowerment invites us to examine where we place value and how we navigate the intersection of choice and identity. In doing so, it challenges us to appreciate the profound impact that autonomy has on our sense of self and community. As this conversation evolves, it becomes evident that empowerment is not an end goal but a continuous journey requiring constant engagement, reflection, and action from each of us.

In the broader context of women's rights and social movements, redefining empowerment finds its power in bridging individual experiences with collective advocacy. Each action that aligns with personal body autonomy adds to the growing tapestry of empowerment. This collective momentum brings strength and validation to personal narratives, reinforcing the belief that individual choices contribute to larger societal transformations.

Let's nurture this dialogue and foster a world where empowerment and body autonomy are seen not as exceptions but as the norm. The ongoing redefinition of empowerment reminds us that change is possible, and every small step taken in pursuit of autonomy is a step towards a more equitable future. As we carry this message forward, let's commit to actively shaping a world that honors choice, celebrates diversity, and champions the fundamental right to comfort and self-determination for all.

Personal Freedom Narratives

Empowerment and body autonomy often find their most vivid expressions through personal freedom narratives. These narratives, deeply rooted in individual experiences, illuminate the profound impact of choosing comfort and embracing body autonomy, especially within the context of the no-bra movement. Every story is a testament to personal courage, a challenge to societal norms, and a declaration of one's right to exist comfortably and confidently in one's skin.

The journey towards personal freedom can begin in the most ordinary settings: a morning routine interrupted by the discomfort of an underwire or an ordinary workday where breathing feels constrained. For many women, the decision to go braless isn't just about physical comfort; it's a rebellion against the silent societal decrees that dictate how feminine bodies should be presented. Choosing not to wear a bra, for a woman who has grown up absorbing messages about modesty and propriety, can be an act of profound personal liberation.

Consider the story of Claire, a marketing executive in her thirties, who spent years conforming to conventional office attire. For her, the introduction to the no-bra movement felt like shedding an invisible layer of societal expectations. Initially nervous about breaking "dress code norms," she soon realized that her colleagues, both male and female, cared little about her choice—or rather, her newfound confidence overshadowed any curiosities they might have had. Claire's story highlights how assertive comfort choices can create ripples within professional environments, influencing others to question and potentially shed their discomforts too.

Other stories emerge from more public realms, where personal decisions intertwine with advocacy. Take Ava, a student activist who realized that going braless could be both a personal relief and a political statement. For Ava, participating in rallies and discussions about women's rights while embracing her body as it naturally is, exemplified her belief that women's comfort shouldn't be compromised for appearances or outdated social sensibilities. Her journey underscores how personal freedom narratives can inspire collective movements, encouraging others to redefine empowerment through their lenses.

However, stepping into such personal freedoms is not without its challenges. In many cultures, the choice to forgo a bra is met with skepticism or judgment, often reflective of deeply ingrained gender norms. For families and communities conditioned to view a woman's appearance through a prism of traditional values, the decision can evoke more discomfort than liberation. Yet, in overcoming these barriers, personal narratives gain strength, illustrating the tension between individual autonomy and collective expectations.

Interestingly, stories that unfold in more liberal settings often depict different challenges. Here, the struggle might not be about confronting external criticism but rather about navigating one's internalized biases. Many women report a profound transition period where learned insecurities surface, as years of being told how a 'proper' silhouette should look can be hard to unlearn. In these journeys, the narrative of personal freedom is as much about emotional resilience as it is about physical liberation. It's an ongoing process of reeducating the mind to view one's body not as an object to fit into societal molds but as a vessel worthy of comfort and care.

Furthermore, these narratives are not restricted to women alone. They resonate with anyone who challenges rigid dress norms to prioritize their comfort. Stories from non-binary and transgender individuals emphasize how body autonomy intertwines with gender identity, showcasing how choosing comfort can be an essential part of affirming one's true self. These accounts add layers to the discourse, highlighting the universality of the desire for bodily comfort across diverse identities.

As the no-bra movement gains momentum, social media becomes a powerful platform for individuals to share their personal freedom narratives. Online spaces like blogs, vlogs, and forums offer safe havens where stories resonate globally, allowing them to transcend borders and cultures. These digital narratives play a crucial role in reinforcing community support and debunking myths, making the movement more accessible to those hesitant to take the first step in their journey toward body autonomy.

In this way, personal freedom narratives are not just stories; they're lifelines. They uplift, reassure, and empower, allowing individuals to see that their feelings of discomfort are valid and that the pursuit of personal liberation is commendable. Each narrative weaves into a larger tapestry illustrating the varied experiences of those who dare to redefine the terms of their comfort and, by extension, their personal empowerment.

These narratives also serve as living historical records. They capture a cultural shift towards embracing natural body shapes and encourage future generations to appreciate their bodies on their terms. Stories allow individuals to own their narrative, positioning them as active agents in shaping societal norms rather than passive adherents.

Personal freedom narratives are raw, intimate, and often profoundly transformative. They capture the essence of choosing liberation over convention and highlight the personal empowerment that emerges from the simple, yet radical, act of embracing one's body as it is. As more individuals step forward to share their truths, these narratives will continue to inspire, motivate, and pave the way for a freer, more inclusive understanding of body autonomy.

Chapter 11:
The Science of Comfort

The science behind comfort is both a physical and psychological exploration—a journey of understanding how the smallest details, like fabric and fit, can influence a woman's state of being. While the sensation of donning a bra can feel akin to an embrace for some, others experience it as an act of restraint, a daily tug against their sense of liberation. Scientifically, comfort is more than just a feeling; it's a tangible element impacting our bodily functions, emotions, and mental clarity. Psychologically, the autonomy to choose comfort over conformity is liberating, sending a powerful message to oneself about self-worth and self-acceptance. By delving into the nuances of what constitutes comfort, we're invited to redefine what embodies our personal peace and challenge the structures—social or synthetic—that impede it. Tapping into this understanding inspires us to prioritize personal well-being over societal dictate, creating a landscape where women can embrace comfort unapologetically.

Understanding Physical Comfort

In a world where societal constructs often dictate what a woman should wear, understanding physical comfort has emerged as a crucial element in the conversation about body autonomy and the no-bra movement. Our bodies innately seek comfort, a fundamental aspect of human experience that extends beyond mere physical sensations. It integrates our emotional states, social interactions, and even cultural norms to form a comprehensive understanding of what comfort truly means. Physical comfort isn't just about choosing what's easy; it's an essential empowering tool in reclaiming one's own body.

Physical comfort begins with acknowledging the body's needs. At the core, it's about feeling at ease without the constraints or discomfort imposed by conventional clothing or societal expectations. For centuries, women have been told how to dress, often prioritizing aesthetics or social conformity over individual comfort. The result? A pervasive sense of unease and disconnection from one's own physicality. In the grand scheme, understanding physical comfort challenges these entrenched norms, advocating for choices that prioritize personal well-being.

It's important to note that comfort is subjective. What feels liberating for one person might not be the same for another. This subjectivity highlights the necessity of self-awareness and personal choice. For some, wearing a bra could offer a sense of security and structure. For others, it represents restriction. Understanding physical comfort calls for this recognition of personal autonomy—allowing women to listen to their bodies and choose accordingly, without the looming cloud of judgment.

Exploring physical comfort also involves diving into the technical aspects that contribute to discomfort. Bras, for example, designed with underwires and tight straps, can cause physical strain. Studies have shown that tight bras might restrict lymphatic flow, potentially leading to health issues. Recognizing the body's signals—soreness, restricted breathing, or discomfort—is crucial in identifying and mitigating unnecessary physical stress. This knowledge empowers women to make informed decisions about what they wear.

In examining comfort, we also consider how modern innovations are shaping our understanding. The rise of athleisure and comfort-focused clothing lines reflects a shifting trend. These advancements challenge the status quo by offering alternatives that merge style with ease. As the demand grows, so does the market for innovative designs that focus on adaptability to various body types and needs. This evolution indicates a broader shift towards valuing individual comfort over external validation.

Physical comfort also transcends the personal and becomes social when considering how societal expectations influence personal choices. The pressure to conform to a conventional image often complicates a woman's day-to-day choices, overshadowing her comfort with perceived societal acceptance. Here, understanding physical comfort means questioning and actively resisting societal norms that suggest discomfort is acceptable as long as the woman looks "appropriate."

Moreover, physical comfort is linked intricately with emotional comfort. Body autonomy allows individuals to feel more at peace with their choices, strengthening self-trust and self-expression. When a woman opts for comfort-centered clothing, she's not just embracing a physical state but also making a statement about how she chooses to perceive her body and her self-worth. In this sense, physical comfort becomes a pathway to emotional liberation.

In the broader social dialogue, promoting physical comfort celebrates uniqueness and diversity, breaking away from one-size-fits-all standards. Every woman's body is distinct, and so are her comfort requirements. Affirming these differences as strengths—rather than inconveniences to be molded into a singular ideal—is crucial for fostering a culture of acceptance and support.

As conversations around the no-bra movement continue to gain traction, they invite an honest examination of historical practices that prioritize discomfort for the sake of beauty or decency. By understanding physical comfort, society can challenge outdated perceptions, opening the door to diverse expressions of femininity that honor personal comfort as a fundamental right.

By embracing physical comfort as a guiding principle, women can move towards a future where their choices aren't dictated by external standards but are instead reflections of personal needs and desires. This future celebrates women's agency and respects their decisions over arbitrary social pressures. As this movement grows, it stands as a testament to the power of choosing comfort, enhancing self-esteem, and promoting a harmonious relationship with one's body.

In the end, understanding physical comfort is more than just a movement; it is a fundamental human right that empowers and inspires women to reclaim their autonomy. It prompts a collective reimagining of comfort, advocating for systems and attitudes that put the individual first. And as society embraces this change, it will undoubtedly move closer to a place where comfort, both physical and emotional, is recognized as an irrefutable aspect of personal freedom.

Psychological Aspects of Comfort

In understanding the science of comfort, we must first delve into the psychological realm, exploring how our mental and emotional states intertwine with our pursuit of comfort. At its core, comfort is a subjective experience; it is deeply personal and inherently tied to our perceptions and emotions. The way we perceive comfort is influenced by a myriad of factors, including cultural norms, personal preferences, and past experiences. Each individual's comfort journey is unique, shaped by their own psychological landscape.

The psychology of comfort often begins with our childhood experiences. Many of us learn about comfort through environmental cues and familial interactions. These early experiences create a blueprint that influences our adult choices, whether it's the clothes we wear, the spaces we inhabit, or the societal norms we choose to challenge. For women, these imprinted narratives often intersect with broader societal expectations about femininity and appearance.

One of the most profound psychological aspects of comfort is the role of body image in our self-perception. The No-Bra movement challenges traditional beauty standards, inviting women to redefine what comfort means on an individual level. Moving away from restrictive clothing, such as a bra, can be a radical act of self-acceptance, fostering a positive body image. This shift encourages women to embrace their natural forms, relinquishing societal pressures that dictate the ideal female silhouette.

Self-perception is significantly influenced by external validation. Women often find comfort in approval from peers, family, and society at large. However, the No-Bra movement exemplifies how seeking internal validation can lead to a more profound sense of comfort. It challenges women to prioritize their own feelings of ease and well-being over societal expectations. This internal shift can be empowering, allowing women to develop a stronger sense of self-identification that isn't contingent on the opinions of others.

Mindfulness and self-awareness also play crucial roles in the psychological aspects of comfort. Mindfulness encourages individuals to listen to their bodies, understanding their unique comfort needs without judgment or comparison. By fostering self-awareness, women can make choices based on how they truly feel, rather than what they think they should feel according to societal norms. This approach not only enhances personal comfort but can also lead to improved mental health outcomes.

Moreover, emotional resilience is another psychological factor linked to comfort. The journey towards embracing comfort, particularly in contexts like the No-Bra movement, requires resilience against potential backlash and criticism. Developing emotional strength supports individuals in resisting external pressures, thus enabling them to maintain their personal comfort choices in the face of societal scrutiny.

Community support and shared experiences can significantly bolster psychological comfort. When women unite around movements that champion comfort and body autonomy, they create a collective resilience. This community provides a support network that offers affirmation, shared experiences, and encouragement, strengthening each member's resolve to embrace their comfort journey. It becomes a psychologically nurturing space where women can explore and articulate their comfort needs without fear or shame.

Personal identity and empowerment are closely linked to comfort. As women explore what true comfort means to them, they often uncover deeper layers of personal empowerment. Choosing to prioritize personal comfort can be a liberating decision, fostering a sense of agency and control over one's body. This empowerment facilitates a clearer expression of personal identity, unencumbered by the strictures of societal expectations.

Ultimately, the psychological aspects of comfort encompass a journey towards self-discovery and acceptance. It's about unwinding the complex layers of societal influence and personal history to reach a place of genuine self-comfort. This journey reflects a broader societal shift towards valuing individual experience and mental well-being, challenging us to rethink how we define and pursue comfort in our lives.

In a world where traditional norms have long dictated how comfort is perceived and experienced, the psychological aspects of this journey become a roadmap towards both personal and collective liberation. As women continue to question and reshape what comfort means, they pave the way for future generations to live with a deeper and more authentic sense of self-comfort and empowerment.

Chapter 12:
Common Myths and Misconceptions

Throughout the ongoing journey of the No-Bra movement, several myths and misconceptions have clouded public understanding and stifled open dialogue. One of the most prevalent myths suggests that forgoing a bra inherently leads to physical discomfort or sagging, despite emerging research challenging these outdated beliefs. Others inaccurately associate not wearing a bra with a lack of professionalism or femininity, ignoring the diversity of modern identities that embrace choice and body autonomy. These misconceptions are often rooted in societal norms that prioritize conventional appearances over genuine comfort and personal freedom. By engaging critically with these myths, we can begin dismantling the barriers they create, empowering individuals to choose what's best for their bodies and lives. Recognizing and addressing these common misunderstandings is crucial in promoting a culture that values authenticity and respects personal choices, contributing to a broader movement toward body positivity and self-acceptance.

Debunking Popular Myths

The No-Bra movement, like any social trend that challenges the status quo, is surrounded by a host of myths and misconceptions. These myths often serve to undermine the legitimate concerns of those advocating for comfort and body autonomy. Myths persist because they are fueled by outdated societal norms and misinformation that many accept without critical examination. Debunking these myths is crucial for understanding the true intentions and motivations of the movement. Let's dig into some of the most prevalent falsehoods and set the record straight.

One widespread myth is the idea that not wearing a bra is purely an act of rebellion against societal norms and offers no real benefits. However, many women choose to go braless for a host of personal reasons that contribute to their well-being. For some, it's all about the comfort that comes with ditching the restrictive confines of a bra, allowing for better circulation and less pressure on the skin. Others find that going braless aligns with their values of embracing natural body shapes and rejecting beauty standards that dictate how a woman's body should appear. It's not always about making a statement; sometimes, it's about feeling good in one's own skin.

Closely tied to this is the misconception that bra-free living is inherently unkempt or unprofessional. Fashion and professional standards are evolving, and the era when a woman's worth was tied to how closely she adhered to rigid dress codes is fading. Many workplaces are beginning to embrace diversity in appearance and prioritize skills over attire. Moreover, fashion has seen a rise in garments designed to support a braless lifestyle without sacrificing style or professionalism. This shift challenges the notion that professionalism requires a tightly structured wardrobe.

Another myth suggests that the No-Bra movement is simply a fad driven by a small group of radicals or celebrities seeking attention. While public figures can help spread awareness, the movement has roots that stretch back decades and involve a wide array of diverse voices advocating for women's rights and comfort across age, race, and socioeconomic backgrounds. These advocates see the movement not as a fleeting trend but as part of an ongoing conversation about body autonomy and self-expression. In truth, the movement gains strength from the collective experiences of everyday women who find solidarity and empowerment in making choices that feel right for their bodies.

One cannot overlook the scientific myths surrounding bra usage and breast health. A persistent myth claims that going braless causes breast sagging. Yet, research offers a more nuanced look at the relationship between bras and breast health, with some studies even suggesting that long-term bra usage might contribute to weaker breast tissue over time. It's essential to recognize that sagging is a natural result of aging and genetic factors, not simply a consequence of not wearing a bra. By confronting these scientific fallacies, we promote an informed dialogue based on evidence rather than fear.

Also prevalent is the belief that bras are a necessity for preventing breast pain. While some women do find bras alleviate discomfort, it's not universally true. The source of breast pain can vary widely, and for some, a bra exacerbates rather than relieves the issue. It's crucial to acknowledge that comfort is subjective, and what works for one person may not work for another. By dispelling the myth that bras are the only solution to breast pain, we empower individuals to explore alternative options that suit their unique needs, such as various types of clothing or lifestyle changes.

The myth that a woman's worth is tied to her adherence to societal norms about appearance is perhaps the most damaging. This belief not only limits personal freedom but also perpetuates a culture where judgment based on physical appearance is normalized. Shifting the narrative to focus on empowerment and self-worth, irrespective of societal expectations, dismantles these harmful ideas and creates space for body positivity and acceptance. This transformative perspective promotes a culture where individuals are celebrated for who they are, not what they look like.

Finally, there's a misconception that participation in the No-Bra movement negates the choice or desire to wear a bra for specific circumstances or personal preference. Advocates for body autonomy emphasize the freedom to choose, recognizing that empowerment comes in different forms. For some, wearing a bra might enhance confidence in particular settings, or they may simply prefer the structure it provides at times. The point is not to universally reject bras but to underscore the importance of personal choice and the right to make decisions about one's body without external pressure.

In debunking these popular myths, we clear the path for a broader acceptance of diverse choices regarding body autonomy. The No-Bra movement, far from being an act of rebellion without reason, is a testament to the evolving conversation about personal comfort, empowerment, and the pressure to conform. As we move forward, understanding and dispelling myths creates room for more nuanced dialogues. Such conversations champion individual expression and pave the way for a society where choice is celebrated and respected. Each myth unraveled ignites a deeper understanding and promotes genuine empowerment.

Public Misunderstandings

For many, the No-Bra movement is mired in misconceptions that cloud its goals and impact. These misunderstandings often stem from deeply ingrained cultural narratives about femininity, modesty, and societal norms. One common notion is that going braless is merely an extension of youthful rebellion or a trend perpetuated by celebrities seeking attention. In truth, the movement is far more nuanced, intertwining deeply personal choices with broader societal implications.

The act of choosing not to wear a bra is often mistakenly reduced to frivolity or fashion trends. Yet, for countless women, it's a profound statement about autonomy and comfort. Many misunderstand this choice as being indicative of a woman's desire to make a political statement or to simply follow the latest trend. On the contrary, for many, it is simply about personal comfort and the desire to live unhindered by societal expectations.

Critics sometimes propose that the No-Bra movement is a rejection of femininity. This misunderstanding arises from the traditional association of bras with the ideal feminine figure. Bras, in many societies, are seen as essential components of female identity. Choosing not to wear one can then be misinterpreted as rejecting womanhood itself, when the reality is quite the opposite. It's a celebration of authentic self-expression, allowing women to embrace their bodies as they are.

There is also a persistent myth that women who choose to go without a bra are primarily doing so for the attention of others, particularly men. This assumption not only objectifies women but also disregards the movement's intrinsic value of personal freedom. The No-Bra movement isn't about seeking validation or approval; it is about asserting body autonomy in a world that often prioritizes others' comfort over one's own.

Another common misunderstanding revolves around the belief that going braless is universally uncomfortable or even harmful. Despite some lingering myths about the necessity of bras for physical health, recent studies suggest that wearing a bra may not offer significant benefits for breast health and can sometimes even contribute to discomfort or poor posture. These findings challenge the narrative that bras are an indispensable aspect of a woman's daily attire.

There's also a frequent concern about professionalism and societal norms, suggesting that not wearing a bra is inappropriate or disrespectful in certain settings. However, this mindset is slowly changing as conversations about women's rights and body autonomy become more mainstream. Over time, what was once deemed unprofessional may come to be seen as a legitimate choice in self-presentation.

Public misunderstandings are further fueled by sensationalist media portrayals and the reduction of the movement to sound bites and clickbait headlines. Media portrayal often simplifies the plight and intentions of women in the movement, overshadowing their genuine pursuit of comfort and autonomy. By exploring these narratives in greater depth, we can begin to appreciate the broader societal shifts that the movement represents.

While some view the No-Bra movement as an affront to traditional values, others see it as an integral part of the broader push for women's rights and body positivity. The movement is about more than just bras—it's about dismantling decades-old norms and creating a space where clothing choices do not equate to personal worth or societal value. It's part of an ongoing dialogue about how clothes and freedom of choice intertwine.

Public misunderstandings often stem from fear of the familiar dissolving into the unknown. The choice to go braless challenges the status quo and asks society to reconsider its long-standing assumptions about femininity and propriety. By examining these myths, we invite a deeper understanding not just of the movement, but of the transformative power of personal choice.

Ultimately, clearing up these misconceptions will take time, effort, and ongoing dialogue. Through education and an open exchange of ideas, society can begin to embrace a more inclusive understanding that honors each woman's right to choose what best suits her body and lifestyle. Public understanding of the No-Bra movement will improve as more people engage in meaningful discussions and listen to those who choose comfort over conformity.

Chapter 13:
Steps Towards Personal Comfort

In a world that often dictates what women should wear to fit societal standards, taking steps toward personal comfort becomes an empowering act of self-liberation. The journey away from wearing bras isn't just about ridding oneself of an undergarment; it's about embracing a freedom that prioritizes well-being over imposed norms. Choosing comfort-conscious clothing means listening to one's own body and needs, selecting fabrics that breathe and forms that allow for natural movement, cultivating a wardrobe that feels like a second skin rather than armor. Transitioning away from constrictive garments could start with small adjustments, like opting for looser fits or experimenting with supportive but non-restrictive alternatives. The shift encourages women to take ownership of their bodies, fostering a daily routine wrapped in personal choice and authenticity. This is a critical step, not only towards individual comfort but also in redefining collective standards of beauty and autonomy. Every decision made in favor of comfort is a step toward personal empowerment, challenging outdated beliefs and inspiring a more accepting culture. It's about crafting a reality where women can move freely and confidently, embodying a true sense of their own comfort and choice.

Choosing Comfort-Conscious Clothing

Embarking on the journey towards personal comfort is an intimate decision that speaks to the heart of self-care and self-expression. At its core, the selection of comfort-conscious clothing reflects not just an aesthetic choice but a deeper commitment to honoring one's body. This section delves into the art and science of choosing garments that promote ease and liberation, rejecting the societal dictates that have long restricted freedom and comfort for women.

Clothing is more than fabric sewn together; it's a statement. It's a silent declaration of who you are and what you value. For decades, women have been conditioned to prioritize appearance over ease, often at the expense of their own comfort. High heels, corsets, and underwire bras are just a few examples of clothing items that historically have been favored for aesthetic appeal despite their discomfort. It's time to redefine how we perceive fashion, prioritizing garments that celebrate natural shapes and enhance daily comfort.

When choosing comfort-conscious clothing, it's essential to begin with understanding what comfort means to you personally. For some, it's about soft, breathable fabrics that move with the body. For others, it means loose-fitting styles that don't constrict. Begin by assessing the clothing you already own—identify pieces that you reach for time and again because they offer the freedom your body craves. Notice the patterns, fabrics, and fits that make those items your favorites, as they are the keys to understanding your style of comfort.

Fabric choice plays a crucial role in comfortable attire. Natural fabrics like cotton, bamboo, and linen often offer breathability and softness that synthetic materials may lack. These textiles allow the skin to breathe, reducing sweat and discomfort. They move with you, adapting to the day's demands rather than working against them. Moreover, sustainability benefits often accompany natural fabrics, aligning your comfort with an eco-conscious lifestyle.

A significant part of this process involves examining how clothing fits. For many, the dilemma isn't just about going braless; it's also about finding clothing that accommodates and celebrates the natural body shape. The fashion industry has often ignored this, tailoring designs for a specific, often unrealistic body type. It's essential to search for brands and designers who challenge this norm, providing diverse sizing options without compromising on style.

While it's tempting to think that trends dictate our wardrobes, it's empowering to develop a personal style based on authenticity and comfort. This doesn't mean rejecting fashion altogether. Instead, it's about integrating pieces that align with individual comfort and make you feel both physically at ease and mentally empowered. This approach maintains your connection to fashion while prioritizing your own wellbeing.

The no-bra movement illuminates one significant aspect of this clothing journey. By challenging the necessity of bras, women around the world are questioning preconceived notions of what is deemed appropriate attire. This is an invitation to re-evaluate wardrobe staples, scrutinizing each item for its comfort contribution. For those starting this transition, prioritizing tops with supportive designs and natural chest support can offer reassurance and confidence.

Adopting a comfort-first approach inevitably intersects with empowerment. It's about taking back control over one's body and choices, one piece of clothing at a time. This conscious shift demonstrates autonomy, refusing to submit to the arbitrary rules of fashion that have historically dictated discomfort as a norm. It's about ensuring that each garment you wear contributes positively to how you experience the world around you.

Exploration is a key part of this journey. With countless fashion retailers and emerging designers advocating for body positivity and comfort, the landscape is ripe for discovery. Many brands are finally listening to the voices demanding change, broadening their offerings to celebrate all body types with inclusive sizing and adaptable styles. Seek out these advocates of change, and let their pieces guide your journey towards a more comfortable wardrobe.

In pursuit of comfort, reflect on how these choices impact your daily life. Consider how the right clothing can transform not just how you feel physically but how you perceive yourself in social settings. When clothing fits right and feels good, the confidence it brings is undeniable. It's an act of self-love, reaffirming the right to feel at ease in one's own skin.

As you choose comfort-conscious clothing, embrace the freedom to experiment. Blend practicality with personal expression, allowing your wardrobe to evolve alongside your understanding of comfort. Fashion isn't static; it's a canvas that evolves with time and attitude. By prioritizing comfort, you craft a narrative that aligns with core values, setting a powerful example for others.

Ultimately, the journey towards comfort-conscious clothing is deeply personal. It's an ongoing exploration that encourages women to discard societal pressures and embrace their bodies with respect and compassion. It's a path toward authenticity, where comfort and empowerment walk hand in hand, reshaping the tapestry of women's lives one liberating choice at a time.

Tips for Transitioning Away from Bras

The journey towards personal comfort in stepping away from conventional bra use is deeply individual. It's not just about ditching a piece of clothing; it's about embracing a newfound sense of self and autonomy. Some women might find it freeing from the first day, while others might need a bit of time and experimentation to get there. Whether it's a leap you've been hesitant to take or a transition you're eagerly anticipating, understanding both the practical and emotional elements of this change is essential.

Start by acknowledging the psychological aspects of this transition. Many women have been conditioned to see bras as essential elements of their wardrobe. That's why the shift begins in the mind. Engage in self-reflection about why you feel the need to wear a bra. Is it comfort, social expectations, or simply habit? By identifying these motivations, you can address and challenge them.

Comfort is key. Consider trying out bralettes or soft, stretchy tops that offer gentle support without the rigidity of underwires. These alternatives can help ease the transition, providing comfort and a sense of security while your body adjusts. Remember, the goal is not about a complete elimination of support, but finding what feels best for you. Everyone's comfort level is different, and experimenting with different options can help you discover what you prefer.

Next, dive into fabric and fashion choices. Certain materials might feel more comfortable against your skin, offering support without restriction. Look for natural fibers like cotton or bamboo, which are breathable and gentle. In the same way, loose-fitting shirts or layered outfits can provide a sense of protection and confidence as you navigate your bra-free journey in public spaces. Explore how these fashion choices can align with your personal style while ensuring comfort.

It's also helpful to think about breast health during this transition. There's often a debate regarding the health benefits or risks associated with ditching bras, and it's essential to consult credible, scientific sources or a trusted health professional for advice tailored to your body. Understanding how your body responds can alleviate worries and support your confidence in making the switch.

Social dynamics can play a significant role in this transition. It's natural to feel self-conscious about the reactions of others, but remember that societal norms are ever-evolving. Find a community or support group that shares your views on comfort and body autonomy.

Engaging with others who have walked the same path can provide encouragement and practical tips, solidifying the idea that you're not alone in this shift. Sharing experiences can build camaraderie and strength over personal choice.

Develop a personal narrative that celebrates your choice rather than justifies it. Base your transition on empowerment and body positivity. Remind yourself daily why you're choosing this route and allow that to reaffirm your decisions. Crafting a positive mindset around your choice can be incredibly liberating, reinforcing that your body is your own and you decide what comfort means.

For those concerned about how this might affect their professional life, understand your workplace policy regarding dress codes. If concerns arise, discreet and comfortable options exist that accommodate different environments without compromising on your ideals. Remember, professional attire does not necessitate discomfort, and advocating for personal comfort is increasingly respected in today's evolving workplace environments.

As you transition, be patient with yourself. This process is not a one-size-fits-all solution and may involve trial and error. What's most important is that you're making this decision for yourself, embracing your comfort needs, and stepping into an era of personal empowerment. The act of transitioning away from bras is not just about rejecting discomfort; it's about choosing authenticity and self-acceptance in a world largely dictated by external expectations. Embrace the journey toward personal comfort, celebrating each step as a testament to your strength and individualism.

Chapter 14:
The Future of the No-Bra Movement

The future of the No-Bra movement is a tapestry of diverse threads weaving together a new narrative of women's empowerment and comfort. As more women embrace body autonomy and challenge outdated norms, we see emerging trends that signal a shift in cultural attitudes. Young people, empowered by social media and digital platforms, are leading the charge, sharing their stories and influencing public perception like never before. This movement is not just about personal comfort but also a profound statement on choice and self-acceptance. It's inspiring to witness how these shifts are resonating across generations, sparking dialogues that elevate the conversation beyond personal preference and into the realm of collective empowerment. With fashion designers increasingly casting aside traditional bra designs in favor of comfort and style, and the influence of global perspectives adding richness to the dialogue, the No-Bra movement is poised to shape a future where every individual feels empowered to make choices for themselves. This is a future where comfort and choice are celebrated, and where the liberation from constraints is both a personal and universal journey. The path forward is not just about dismantling norms but building a new landscape where women's comfort is seen as a foundational right rather than an optional luxury.

Emerging Trends

The trajectory of the No-Bra movement is akin to a powerful river winding through the landscape of society, sculpting new paths and reshaping old foundations. As societal attitudes evolve towards greater gender equality, body autonomy, and inclusivity, there's a distinct shift towards embracing personal comfort and authentic self-expression. The movement isn't just about discarding a piece of clothing; it's about redefining how women perceive themselves and are perceived in the world.

One notable trend is the rapid rise of digital communities and social media platforms as spaces of empowerment. Online, women share their stories, support one another, and challenge entrenched beauty standards. These communities amplify voices that encourage confidence without conforming to traditional expectations. The internet has also fostered a proliferation of educational content, where discussions about bra usage's health implications mingle with personal testimonials, creating a rich tapestry of experience-sharing and mutual empowerment.

As these discussions unfold in the digital realm, they're also impacting real-world practices and consumer behavior. The fashion industry is increasingly acknowledging a demand for garments that don't necessitate the wearing of a bra. Designers are innovating with supportive clothing that champions natural forms and encourages comfort without sacrificing style. Some brands have committed to more inclusive sizing and designs that cater to a diverse array of body shapes, embodying a shift towards ethical and consumer-centered fashion.

Technology's role in shaping this movement can't be understated. Innovative textile engineering is giving rise to new fabrics and designs that offer support without constraint. This blend of comfort and functionality is punctuating the fashion sector with possibilities that align with the No-Bra movement's ethos. As technology advances, it's likely we'll see even more exciting developments that marry innovation with the core value of freeing female bodies from unnecessary discomfort.

Cultural attitudes are another pivotal factor. There's a growing acceptance of varied body types and an understanding that comfort should not be gender-exclusive. Initiatives promoting body positivity are integrating with the No-Bra movement, strengthening its potential to bring about deeper change. As a result, the narrative around bras is evolving from one of necessity to preference, where individual choice becomes the guiding principle.

Simultaneously, generational shifts bring fresh perspectives. Younger generations seem more willing to challenge long-held beliefs about appearance and gender roles. Many Gen Z women, having grown up in a culture that increasingly values diversity and inclusion, are at the forefront of questioning why bras are considered essential. For them, going without is not always a statement of rebellion but a simple embrace of choice and personal comfort.

However, it's crucial to recognize the diversity within the movement. While some lean towards complete bra rejection, others seek a balance where different occasions prompt different choices in comfort and support. This duality of choice respects individual preferences and lifestyle demands without imposing a singular view of empowerment. It's this multiplicity of paths that reinforces the underlying message: every woman's comfort journey is uniquely her own.

Moreover, there's an increasing intersection between the No-Bra movement and environmental concerns. Minimalism and sustainability are powerful allies in this context, advocating for fewer clothing items and a lesser environmental footprint. Many participants in the movement are also conscientious about the implications of consumerism, opting for quality of life over volume of goods. This mindfulness extends to challenging the 'disposable fashion' mentality, thereby encouraging sustainability through the lens of personal comfort choices.

The workplace is another domain seeing shifts due to these unfolding trends. Corporate policies are increasingly scrutinized for their roles in dictating women's attire, leading some organizations to reevaluate dress codes in favor of more inclusive and accommodating guidelines. While there remains progress to be made, this gradual change in work environments is symptomatic of larger societal developments that are asking: What does professionalism look like when comfort is factored in?

It's clear that as we move forward, the No-Bra movement will continue to influence broader discussions around autonomy and freedom. Encouraging a mindset that values comfort on one's terms, it symbolizes a new era where women's bodies aren't just celebrated for their variety but are honored for their needs. As we progress, these emerging trends carve out a promising path, illustrating how individual choices can reshape societal norms for the better.

Ultimately, the No-Bra movement is a testament to how powerful conjoint voices can be in transforming personal decisions into collective momentum for change. The momentum is not just about bras; it's about embracing every facet of individuality and comfort in defiance of past limitations. As these trends continue to emerge, they assert that when it comes to our bodies, there truly is no 'one size fits all' mandate.

Influences on the Next Generation

As the No-Bra Movement continues to evolve, it's crucial to understand how it influences younger generations. At its core, the movement advocates for comfort and personal choice in clothing, challenging societal norms that have long dictated what women should wear. This chapter delves into how the movement's principles are being absorbed by today's youth and shaping their understanding of comfort, body autonomy, and societal expectations.

The No-Bra Movement's impact on younger people starts with education. As discussions about body positivity and women's rights become more prevalent in schools and media, young people are being introduced to alternative narratives about body image and comfort. These conversations encourage them to question traditional standards and to embrace their bodies as they are. In a way, they're learning to prioritize their own comfort over imposed norms, a significant shift from past generations.

Moreover, the portrayal of the No-Bra Movement and related ideas in popular culture plays a pivotal role. Social media platforms have become breeding grounds for sharing and disseminating information, including messages from the movement. Influencers and public figures who champion bralessness and body acceptance provide representations that young people can relate to and be inspired by. These digital narratives offer a fresh perspective that aligns more closely with the evolving attitudes of today's youth.

Perhaps one of the most significant influences is the visibility of diverse body types and personal stories shared online. This exposure helps young people develop a more nuanced understanding of beauty, which isn't limited to conventional norms. When celebrities and athletes openly support going braless, it normalizes the concept and subtly instills the message that it's okay to be comfortable in your own skin, regardless of societal standards.

In addition, the rise of environmental consciousness among younger generations can't be ignored. Many young people are aware of the fast fashion industry's impact on the planet and are drawn to sustainable choices. The No-Bra Movement intersects here by promoting minimalism and reducing consumption of unnecessary clothing, including bras that don't align with personal comfort. This alignment with eco-friendly values further strengthens the movement's appeal to environmentally conscious youth.

While the movement encourages individuality, there's a communal aspect too. Online platforms allow young people to connect globally, sharing experiences and supporting each other in their choices. This sense of community empowers them to stand against criticism and encourages others to explore their comfort zones. It builds a sense of solidarity and collective strength, influencing peers positively.

Contrastingly, it's crucial to address the potential pushback that arises from traditional corners. In some cultures, the idea of going braless is still met with resistance, and young people may experience a tug-of-war between progressive ideals and conventional upbringing. Navigating these conflicting messages can be challenging, but it also offers an opportunity for intergenerational dialogue and understanding.

While the movement is gaining traction, its influence isn't uniform across different demographics. Factors such as geographical location, cultural background, and access to information can affect how young people perceive and engage with the No-Bra Movement. Nonetheless, as awareness spreads, these barriers are gradually being dismantled, paving the way for a more inclusive understanding of comfort and autonomy.

The educational system plays a pivotal role in shaping the views of future generations. As schools become more inclusive and open to discussions about body autonomy and personal choice, they provide a fertile ground for young minds to question outdated norms. Curriculums that include lessons on gender equality and body positivity further enhance the impact by providing factual, unbiased information that encourages critical thinking.

With these shifts, young people are increasingly equipped to make informed choices about their bodies and their comfort. They're growing up in an era where personal empowerment is a valued commodity, and this influence will undoubtedly shape how society perceives women's comfort in the future. By championing their right to choose, the next generation is not only embracing the present but also laying the groundwork for future societal transformation.

Furthermore, the role of parents and guardians cannot be underestimated. As they witness the evolution of these movements, adults have the opportunity to influence the next generation positively. By fostering open discussions about comfort, choice, and body image, they can provide a supportive environment that nurtures confidence and understanding. This familial influence is crucial in reinforcing the values promoted by the No-Bra Movement.

As the No-Bra Movement progresses, it's also inspiring new conversations about gender norms and expectations. Young people, who are often at the forefront of challenging normative ideas, see the potential for broader societal changes stemming from this movement. They're beginning to question not only what women are expected to wear but also how clothing choices reflect deeper issues of gender inequality and autonomy.

In light of these influences, it's clear that the No-Bra Movement is sparking a profound transformation in how the next generation perceives personal comfort and societal expectations. As young people continue to embrace these ideals, the movement's impact will resonate beyond the confines of fashion and clothing, fundamentally reshaping conversations about autonomy and self-acceptance.

The future of the No-Bra Movement, as seen through the eyes of youth, is not just about the absence of bras but the presence of choice. It's about instilling a belief in autonomy and fostering a world where decisions about personal comfort are respected and celebrated. This generational shift, inspired by today's advocacy and cultural shifts, promises a future where individuality is embraced and celebrated on a broader scale.

Chapter 15:
Challenging Norms:
A Global Perspective

Around the world, the conversation on body autonomy and comfort isn't just loud—it's transformative. With diverse cultural lenses, many societies are reimagining the norms that have long dictated women's fashion and body image, igniting change that feels both personal and collective. From bustling metropolitan cities to remote villages, international voices are rising, advocating for the freedom to choose comfort over convention. In France, where liberating fashion has historical roots, women boldly embrace the concept of going braless, merging style with empowerment. Meanwhile, in Japan, nuanced discussions on traditional attire and modern comfort reveal a complex tapestry of societal expectations. As we look to Brazil, the fusion of vibrant culture and relaxed norms challenges old perceptions, highlighting the unique ways communities champion personal freedom. Every movement around the globe adds a vital thread to this evolving narrative, illustrating that the quest for comfort transcends borders and fosters a deeper understanding among diverse cultures. This universal shift illustrates an inspiring truth: the journey toward redefining norms is as varied and rich as the landscapes of our world, proving that while paths may differ, the destination of choice and autonomy unites us all.

International Movements

The No-Bra movement is a powerful global phenomenon, stirred by cultural shifts and a drive toward bodily autonomy and comfort. As we zoom out to see this movement through an international lens, we find a mosaic of experiences and activism. Each country hosts a unique dialogue about standards of beauty, societal norms, and personal freedom, influenced by history, politics, and social dynamics.

In France, the birthplace of haute couture, the conversation around the No-Bra movement weaves into the larger fabric of the nation's historical emphasis on fashion and feminism. The French "liberté" ethos, promoting freedom and self-expression, fuels a cultural readiness to challenge restrictive norms. Young women in urban centers like Paris have embraced the movement, seeing it not just as a statement of comfort, but as a declaration of their right to inhabit their bodies as they see fit. In this context, going braless becomes a quiet form of resistance.

Across the Channel, in the United Kingdom, the story unfolds differently. Here, progressive values in metropolitan areas support the movement's visibility. However, this contrasts with traditional perspectives more prevalent in rural areas. Awareness campaigns and festivals celebrating body positivity are bringing attention to the movement, with influential figures using their platforms to normalize the decision to abandon bras. Yet, it continues to grapple with its own cultural conservatisms, making the shift a gradual, layered process.

Moving to the United States, the No-Bra Movement is deeply intertwined with broader social justice causes. Women challenge systems of patriarchy and capitalist structures that commodify the female body. It's a conversation about choice and empowerment, catalyzed by the country's rich history of civil rights activism. The movement here isn't just about not wearing a bra; it's a demand for respect and authority over one's own body, regardless of societal prescriptions.

In Asia, the landscape is diverse and complex, with each nation reflecting its distinct cultural narratives. In Japan, the movement is slowly gaining traction among the younger generation and social media has become a powerful tool to navigate and challenge deeply embedded social norms about femininity and professionalism. Meanwhile, in India, there is a nuanced struggle. Traditional values often clash with modern feminist movements, making the journey towards bra-free acceptance challenging but vital in urban hubs like Mumbai and Delhi.

Latin America's contribution to the dialogue is vibrant and deeply passionate, characterized by grassroots activism and community support networks. In countries like Brazil and Argentina, the No-Bra movement is as much about fighting femicide and gender violence as it is about comfort. The fight for the female body's autonomy intersects with a broader battle for women's rights and gender equality, invigorating public protests and artistic expressions that capture both local and global narratives.

The African continent's response is another dynamic story. In South Africa, for instance, the movement aligns with women's rights activities post-apartheid, fostering discussions about freedom and equality. The choices women make here aren't only influenced by aesthetics but also health, accessibility, and climatic conditions, creating a dialogue that's both intensely personal and community-focused.

Australia and New Zealand present a fascinating study of contrasts, where indigenous perspectives on bodily autonomy add rich layers to the movement. In urban areas, there's an embrace of the No-Bra trend in sync with eco-friendly and minimalist lifestyles. This shift challenges traditional expectations, echoing the wider global call for individual agency and natural comfort.

In the Middle East, the conversation around the No-Bra movement intersects with a complex backdrop of cultural conservatism and burgeoning feminist movements. Countries like Lebanon showcase a more liberal attitude where personal choices are becoming less taboo, while in other parts, the change is slow but evident among younger populations. Online platforms have become a crucial space for dialogue and support, fostering a growing discourse that navigates tradition and modernity.

Despite diverse cultural contexts, a common thread ties these international movements together: the pursuit of comfort intertwined with the assertion of personal rights. Social media has played an instrumental role in uniting these experiences and stories, enabling a cross-pollination of ideas and solidarity among advocates worldwide.

As these movements continue to develop globally, they compellingly underscore the notion that rejecting bras isn't merely a quest for physical comfort, but a symbol of broader shifts towards equality and self-expression. Each region adds its unique voice, further propelling the movement forward and crafting a rich tapestry of global resistance against imposed norms. By understanding the international nuances of the No-Bra movement, we can better appreciate the universal yearnings for freedom, equality, and dignity that drive this movement, inspiring us to consider our own choices within a global continuum.

Global Voices

Throughout history, the world has seen a tapestry of cultural attitudes toward women's bodies and their clothing choices. Today, these attitudes are shifting more rapidly than ever, spurred by voices from every corner of the globe. The no-bra movement, a significant aspect of contemporary feminism and body autonomy, echoes this change. In every culture, women are stepping forward, sharing diverse perspectives, and demanding the freedom to choose what comfort means to them.

There's an assortment of motivations driving women across different nations to embrace or resist the no-bra movement. For instance, in certain Western countries, women's liberation movements have laid a rich groundwork that prompts questioning traditional norms. Here, the movement is more about asserting personal freedom and challenging the status quo. In contrast, in parts of Asia and the Middle East, such movements often intersect more directly with deep-rooted cultural and religious norms, making the act of going braless a radical statement in places steeped in conservative values.

In France, known for its long tradition of fashion-forward thinking and progressive social policies, the no-bra movement intertwines with a cultural appreciation for natural beauty and an ethos of bodily acceptance. French women advocating for bralessness often embrace this choice as a return to authenticity, celebrating the body's natural state and rejecting constructs that dictate otherwise. This standpoint is empowering for many, signaling a rejection of the male gaze and the commercialization of female bodies.

Meanwhile, in Africa, voices from different communities are amplifying the conversation. In some African cultures, where traditional attire does not always require a bra, the transition might seem less about rebellion and more about reclaiming indigenous customs. However, in urban areas where Western attire and ideals are prevalent, going braless can be an act of resistance against neocolonial standards imposed by global fashion industries. African women participating in the global dialogue about bodily autonomy highlight the significance of maintaining cultural identity amidst a homogenizing world.

The narrative in South America offers another unique lens. Here, cultural norms about femininity and body exposure differ considerably across countries. Brazilian women contribute dynamically to the global movement, often drawing from the cultural valorization of the body in contexts like Carnival. This embrace of the body, however, also comes with intense societal scrutiny and pressure to adhere to beauty ideals. The no-bra movement thus coincides with efforts to dismantle these pressures, focusing on celebrating bodies of all shapes and choices.

In India, where societal norms are rapidly evolving, discussions around the no-bra movement are gaining momentum in urban centers. It's a complex issue, as it challenges deeply entrenched views about modesty and femininity. Indian advocates emphasize the importance of personal agency and foster dialogue around comfort and consent, encouraging women to make choices for themselves rather than conforming to societal expectations. This dialogue is critical in a country balancing rapid modernity with traditional norms.

Australian women also add their voices to the global chorus, often highlighting the extremes of Australian climate as a practical consideration for going braless. Here, the movement intersects with a broader lifestyle of informality and comfort that characterizes much of Australian culture. By embracing a braless lifestyle, Australian women reflect the country's larger ethos of easygoing, unfettered living, seamlessly integrating the personal with the cultural.

The Middle East presents a particularly poignant contrast, where cultural sensitivity and societal roles render the no-bra movement both delicate and vital. Women championing this cause often do so anonymously, driven by a desire for bodily autonomy in a context often governed by strict normative codes. Their stories reverberate with courage, insisting on the right to comfort in environments where such topics can quickly become politically charged.

Through all these narratives, common threads persist—the quest for freedom, the celebration of choice, and the challenge to societal norms that prescribe narrow definitions of propriety. Women globally are leveraging digital platforms to exchange ideas, support each other, and forge international networks of solidarity. Social media serves as a crucial conduit, enabling these voices to transcend geographical and cultural barriers, uniting a diverse array of perspectives into a powerful, singular call for change.

Grassroots organizations worldwide are pivotal in amplifying these voices, undertaking local initiatives that educate and empower women about body positivity and personal comfort. From workshops and seminars to online campaigns, these organizations adapt global ideas to fit their local contexts, ensuring that the movement remains inclusive and sensitive to cultural nuances.

As Global Voices merge within the broader framework of the no-bra movement, they invite an equally global audience to reflect on what these choices mean. They compel society to ask what comfort, autonomy, and confidence truly look like in diverse cultural frameworks. How does one generation's challenge to norms inspire the next? How do daily choices accumulate into societal changes? In these questions lies the potential for profound shifts.

The no-bra movement's worldwide reach provides an unprecedented opportunity for cross-cultural exchange and understanding. It highlights how women everywhere, despite differing circumstances and cultural backgrounds, share an intrinsic desire for comfort and autonomy over their bodies. This universal thread unites women across continents, crafting a narrative that is as varied and rich as it is cohesive and strong—a testament to the power of global voices working in tandem to reshape the future.

As these stories continue to weave into an ever-expanding tapestry of women's experiences, they carry an enduring message: comfort is not merely a personal preference but a human right that transcends borders. With every voice that speaks and every choice that supports this movement, the world steps closer to a future where women can take comfort, literally and figuratively, in being exactly who they wish to be.

Chapter 16:
Economic Aspects of
the Bra Industry

In the modern era, the bra industry stands as a colossal entity with deep economic roots and extensive market dynamics, shaping not just livelihoods but also influencing societal norms. The industry's financial clout can't be understated—it's an intricate interplay of consumer demand, marketing, and evolving fashion trends. As the No-Bra movement seeds new thoughts on female autonomy and comfort, it's triggering a significant shift in market patterns. Companies are re-evaluating their strategies as they're forced to adapt, facing potential declines in traditional bra sales while eyeing fresh opportunities in comfort-oriented and innovative undergarment designs. This movement is not just a trend; it's a potential turning point—an economic redefinition driven by women's quest for choice and liberation. It underscores how cultural movements can ripple through markets, compelling industries to innovate or fade. As fashion brands and retailers navigate this evolving landscape, they are being challenged to align economic interests with the growing emphasis on body autonomy and comfort, creating a potential for transformative change.

Bra Market Dynamics

The bra industry, valued in the billions, is a significant component of the global fashion market. It has not only shaped but been shaped by cultural, social, and technological shifts over the decades. With such deep roots in societal norms and identity, this market doesn't just sell a garment, but promises comfort, style, and often, a notion of femininity.

We must ask how an industry evolved to weave itself so intricately into the fabric of women's lives. Historically, bras weren't just for support or modesty; they became symbolic of female identity. As the industry grew in the early 20th century, innovations rushed to meet the expectations and desires of women. The bra's design evolved to reflect the era's idealized femininity—from the flapper-friendly bandeaus of the 1920s to the pointed conical bras of the 1950s.

Yet, market dynamics no longer rely on aesthetic and functional aspects alone. Modern consumers demand more. The rise of the No-Bra movement has redefined comfort and autonomy, leading to fluctuations in traditional bra market dynamics. As more women advocate for body positivity and reject restrictive garments, they challenge brands to rethink product lines and marketing strategies.

Companies face a dual challenge: maintaining traditional customer bases while appealing to a growing segment embracing alternate forms of comfort. Brands have begun to expand their offerings to include bralettes and sport bras, which offer minimal support but maximize comfort. This shift isn't merely an echo of changing fashion trends but a response to consumer advocacy and empowerment movements.

Meanwhile, the No-Bra movement impacts on a macroeconomic scale. It disrupts established supply chains, forces reevaluation of marketing strategies, and even challenges price structures. Established brands must adapt, innovate, or risk becoming obsolete. The industry's adaptability is both a testament to the power wielded by consumer demand and a reflection of shifting cultural landscapes.

The global reach of these dynamics cannot be understated. Consumer behaviors vary widely across regions, influenced by cultural norms and economic conditions. In Asian markets, for instance, there's an emerging appetite for comfort-oriented styles previously categorized as niche. Conversely, some regions in Europe show steadfast loyalty to traditional forms, signaling a complex interplay between tradition and modernity.

Furthermore, e-commerce is reshaping the market in profound ways. Online platforms transcend geographical boundaries, offering consumers a plethora of choices and innovations at their fingertips. This digital shift democratizes access to diverse styles, enabling small, comfort-focused brands to compete alongside industry giants on a global stage.

It's crucial to consider how socioeconomic factors come into play within these market dynamics. The recent global focus on sustainability affects the bra industry as consumers increasingly prefer eco-friendly materials and ethical production practices. Brands are pressured to reevaluate production processes, aiming to reduce environmental impact while maintaining profitability.

In economic terms, as the No-Bra movement gains traction, it introduces new variables into market equations, notably impacting sales forecasts and inventory strategies. Traditional metrics for predicting market trends must be recalibrated to accommodate the unpredictable tides of cultural change. What's evident is that the comfort revolution propels a market once viewed as static into a dynamic future.

The bra market, therefore, stands at a crossroads. It must embrace innovation, sustainability, and inclusivity to thrive. As brands aggregate consumer insights, they must remain agile, recalibrating offerings to align with an ever-evolving conception of comfort, identity, and empowerment. Success hinges on responsiveness to consumer voices, which grow louder and more influential by the day.

Financial Impact of the Movement

The No-Bra movement, a growing trend where many women choose comfort and autonomy over traditional undergarments, has begun to deliver seismic shifts within the bra industry. This change didn't happen overnight; rather, it emerged as an evolving challenge to long-standing societal norms around femininity and fashion. From an economic perspective, the movement has led to both visible tremors and subtle shifts in the bra market, energizing an intriguing dialogue about the financial dynamics that ensue when cultural movements challenge entrenched consumer practices.

Initially, the bra industry regarded the No-Bra movement as a fringe movement, unlikely to impact sales in a significant manner. The industry is large, robust, and quite resilient, with global revenues reaching billions annually. However, as the movement gained momentum through social media and the amplification of body positivity messages, it spurred a noticeable decline in bra sales, particularly within the wired and heavily structured segments. More women began to prioritize comfort over aesthetics, impacting sales figures in traditional product lines that have defined the industry for decades.

What appears as a decline for traditional bras has simultaneously opened new market opportunities. Many companies have responded by expanding their product offerings to include more comfort-oriented options like bralettes, wireless bras, and sports bras. The demand for these alternatives reflects a broader trend towards less restrictive clothing and a shift in consumer mindset from form to function. Forward-thinking companies have adapted their marketing strategies to focus on themes of inclusivity, body positivity, and comfort, aligning with the messages touted by the No-Bra advocates.

Surprisingly, smaller and niche brands have capitalized significantly from this evolution. These companies often have the agility to innovate quickly and can more readily align themselves with niche consumer ideologies. Brands that were once considered minor players in the lingerie market have gained visibility and market share by promoting products that align with modern priorities around comfort and natural body shapes. Start-ups boasting ethical manufacturing processes and body-positive messaging are thriving due to their alignment with the ethos of the No-Bra movement.

Furthermore, this shift has not only affected manufacturing and sales but has also influenced marketing and distribution channels. The conversation around bras is now placed within broader narratives of empowerment and personal choice, transforming marketing tactics. There's been a marked shift towards digital platforms where consumers seek out authentic voices and transparent brand narratives. Influencer marketing, particularly among those who advocate for body positivity and authenticity, has become a powerful channel for reaching the movement's audience.

The financial impact also extends beyond individual brands to include larger economic spheres. The textile and fashion industries have witnessed a diversification in demand for materials previously dictated by the bra industry. This diversification has encouraged innovation in fabric technology, promoting the development of new materials that are both comfortable and environmentally friendly. Supply chains are adjusting to this shift, reflecting broader trends towards sustainability, which further aligns with the ethos of many in the No-Bra movement.

Moreover, the evolving consumer attitude is prompting mainstream retailers to reconsider their place within this new market landscape. Traditionally structured lingerie departments are reimagining their spaces and offerings, integrating more inclusive designs that cater to a wider array of body types and preferences. Retailers that fail to adapt may face reduced foot traffic and sales, as consumers gravitate towards brands that reflect their values and lifestyle preferences.

The economic reverberations are not solely confined to the sale of bras or lingerie. Companies in adjacent industries, including those producing apparel, cosmetics, and personal care, are also adapting to serve an audience that increasingly values combination of comfort, authenticity, and empowerment over traditional standards. These shifts are driving broader conversations about the role of fashion and wellness, fueling innovation and competition within markets influenced by the No-Bra movement.

While it's essential to highlight the economic ripple effects within the industry, one cannot ignore the wider societal implications that accompany these financial shifts. As the industry evolves, it reflects a broader cultural movement towards more inclusive and diverse representations of womanhood. Every dollar redirected from traditional bras challenges outdated norms, fostering a more open dialogue about women's comfort and body autonomy. This economic transition signifies a shift not just in purchasing behavior but in the cultural narrative about what constitutes empowerment and self-expression.

The financial aspect of the No-Bra movement underscores the dynamic interplay between consumer values and market forces. It illustrates the potential for socio-cultural movements to incite economic change and also reflects on how industries can exploit these changes to create new opportunities and drive innovation. As we assess the continual impact of this movement, we see a reinforcement of the idea that economic success and cultural relevance are increasingly intertwined, guiding the evolution of consumer markets in the modern era.

Chapter 17:
The Role of Social Media
in the Movement

In an age where digital presence often shapes societal trends, the No-Bra movement has found a powerful ally in social media. Through platforms like Instagram, Twitter, and TikTok, voices that were once confined to whispers and small gatherings now have a global stage. Young activists use these spaces not just to share personal journeys of liberation but to encourage a communal reevaluation of comfort and autonomy. Hashtags have become rallying cries for body positivity, while viral posts challenge the conventional perceptions of femininity one scroll at a time. Social media's role can't be overstated—it provides a democratic forum where women's stories of empowerment are amplified, fostering an environment ripe for change. Online communities transform the personal into collective momentum, creating a tapestry of support and advocacy that makes the movement impossible to ignore. As these digital threads weave stronger networks, they also unravel long-standing societal norms, inviting everyone to partake in this cultural renaissance.

Online Communities

In the modern era, social media has become an indispensable tool for movements seeking global reach and immediate interaction. The No-Bra Movement, as it evolves, finds a powerful ally in online communities that are reshaping the conversation around women's rights, body positivity, and comfort. Online platforms grant individuals the space to connect, share stories, and find solidarity, amplifying voices that might otherwise be drowned out. Every post, tweet, and shared story contributes to challenging the status quo and promoting body autonomy.

The virtual world thrives on diversity and inclusivity, offering a melting pot of experiences and perspectives. Online communities are uniquely positioned to question traditional roles and promote progressive ideals. They allow people to engage with discussions about the No-Bra Movement in a manner that's both personal and expansive. Participants can exchange ideas, engage in dialogue, and share visual narratives that highlight their journey towards comfort and autonomy. This exchange is crucial in dismantling longstanding societal norms that dictate how women should present themselves to the world.

A significant aspect of these online communities is their ability to foster a sense of belonging. Many women who felt isolated by societal pressures or family expectations find camaraderie and support in these virtual spaces. They become part of a collective voice advocating for the right to choose personal comfort over conforming to outdated standards. Through this shared mission, individuals are empowered to embrace their bodies unapologetically. No longer are they forced to see their choices as acts of rebellion, but rather as expressions of personal freedom and agency.

This shift towards online activism is particularly relevant for younger generations, who often spend a significant portion of their lives digitally connected. The No-Bra Movement's themes of independence and body acceptance resonate deeply with a demographic accustomed to using technology as a means of self-expression. Teens and young adults use social media not only to engage with the movement but also to educate their peers and challenge societal conventions from the ground up. These online discussions are often more impactful than traditional media narratives, mainly because they originate from lived experiences and personal conviction.

The visually-driven nature of platforms like Instagram, TikTok, and Pinterest plays a critical role in normalizing and celebrating the choice to forego bras. Images and videos make abstract ideas more tangible, allowing people to witness the beauty and diversity of bodies in their natural state. What once was seen as a bold statement has become normalized through sheer visibility. As more people share their journeys, others feel inspired and encouraged to embark on their own path towards comfort and authenticity.

Online forums and groups also serve as educational resources. Members post articles, scientific findings, and personal narratives that break down complex topics related to breast health, societal expectations, and the psychology of self-perception. They create safe spaces for inquiry and debate, where questions can be asked without judgment, and information is accessible to all. This democratization of knowledge is vital in dismantling myths and fostering an informed community where each decision is respected.

Importantly, these communities are spaces for digital advocacy. Campaigns like #NoBraDay and #FreeTheNipple have garnered massive traction, drawing attention to the movement's key issues and encouraging broader participation. Hashtags serve as rallying points, effectively organizing and amplifying content across platforms. They symbolize the collective struggle and unity within the movement and have played a pivotal role in shifting public perception and inspiring change at institutional and cultural levels.

It's crucial to recognize how online communities navigate backlash and criticism. Any movement that upends cultural norms inevitably encounters resistance, and the No-Bra Movement is no exception. Online spaces provide a frontline for these debates, where detractors often voice concerns about decorum or appropriateness. However, the resilience displayed within these communities is noteworthy. Activists embrace these challenges, countering misconceptions with facts and real-life experiences. The ability to respond in real time often neutralizes negativity and bolsters the movement's credibility.

The spirit of inclusion extends beyond gender, inviting men into the conversation as allies. Online engagement facilitates these dialogues, where men learn to support the movement, challenge patriarchal norms, and advocate for broadening the definition of comfort and equality. Their involvement signifies a society gradually leaning towards egalitarianism, where movements like No-Bra create ripples of change across gender lines.

It's also essential to acknowledge the potential pitfalls of online communities. While they offer unprecedented opportunities for connection and support, the digital realm is not without its challenges. The risk of misinformation, echo chambers, and cyberbullying are real threats that underscore the need for mindful interaction. Building resilient online communities requires thoughtful moderation and proactive engagement to maintain a respectful and constructive discourse.

Ultimately, the synergy between the No-Bra Movement and online platforms creates a fertile ground for societal transformation. As the movement continues to gain momentum, these virtual connections become invaluable in sustaining awareness and participation. They prove that collective empowerment isn't a distant dream but a tangible reality within reach, underscored by the profound connections formed across borders, cultures, and backgrounds.

The role of online communities in the No-Bra Movement transcends mere support; it signifies a broader cultural shift towards individual autonomy and collective advocacy. As this network of voices expands, it lays down the foundation for future generations to make informed choices free of societal constraints, proving that in unity, there is strength.

Digital Advocacy

In today's hyper-connected world, digital advocacy has become a crucial tool for social movements, transforming the way people engage with and support causes. With the rise of the No-Bra movement, digital advocacy has played an essential role in challenging societal norms and promoting body autonomy. Through social media platforms, online communities have formed, creating spaces for individuals to share experiences, provide support, and advocate for change.

The power of social media lies in its ability to amplify voices that might otherwise go unheard. For the No-Bra movement, this means providing a platform for women to share their stories and highlight the benefits of rejecting restrictive garments. These personal narratives can challenge prevailing stereotypes and offer new perspectives, encouraging others to question established norms. Digital content from blog posts to tweets acts as a catalyst, sparking conversations around topics like body positivity and women's rights, thereby widening the scope of the dialogue beyond traditional boundaries.

Advocacy through digital means democratizes the conversation, making it accessible to anyone with an internet connection. This worldwide access means women across different cultures and socio-economic backgrounds can connect and collaborate. Campaigns often start with a single hashtag, quickly developing into global movements that invite participation, discussion, and change. This level of engagement helps normalize the conversation around female comfort and body autonomy, breaking taboos and altering perceptions in real-time.

While these digital spaces foster community and support, they also face challenges. Algorithms and platform policies can restrict visibility, silencing important messages and limiting reach. Advocacy groups must continuously develop creative and strategic ways to navigate these digital obstacles, using analytical insights to optimize their campaigns. Beyond the platforms themselves, advocates contend with backlash and criticism, which can be a daunting aspect of public online discourse. Yet, this only underscores the importance and potency of digital advocacy in pushing boundaries and effecting change.

Part of digital advocacy's transformative potential lies in its ability to educate and inform. Various educational campaigns provide statistical evidence and personal testimonies to counter myths and misinformation related to the No-Bra movement. Infographics, videos, and interactive content are powerful tools in breaking down complex issues into digestible pieces. This wealth of information encourages individuals to explore their own assumptions and reconsider their views, serving as an entry point into the movement for many.

The role of influencers cannot be ignored in the realm of digital advocacy. When public figures with a large following discuss or align themselves with the No-Bra movement, it can attract attention and lend a certain degree of legitimacy. However, the movement's grassroots nature empowers everyday women to become digital advocates themselves, regardless of their follower count. By participating in campaigns and sharing their journeys, they contribute to a diverse tapestry of voices that collectively drive the movement forward.

Effective digital advocacy hinges on authenticity and relatability. Users resonate with genuine stories and authentic experiences, not manufactured narratives. Thus, many advocates choose to share raw, unfiltered content that captures the realities of choosing comfort over convention. This kind of vulnerability does more than generate engagement; it fosters empathy, a crucial element in building a supportive community and advancing the goals of the No-Bra movement.

Collaborations across different advocacy groups can further amplify messages, weaving the No-Bra movement into the broader tapestry of women's rights issues. Cross-collaboration introduces shared goals and strategies, expanding the reach and impact of digital campaigns. These partnerships bring valuable insights and varying perspectives, enriching the conversation and providing a multifaceted approach to advocacy.

As the movement continues to grow, digital advocacy remains a dynamic and evolving entity. The future holds exciting potential for innovation, with new technologies offering fresh opportunities for engagement. Virtual reality, interactive storytelling, and other technologies could one day redefine how the No-Bra movement interacts with its audience, providing immersive experiences that deepen understanding and support.

In sum, digital advocacy serves as both a sword and a shield in the fight for gender equality and empowerment. It arms advocates with the tools to voice their truths and create ripples of change. This digital dimension of advocacy doesn't just complement the on-the-ground efforts; it revolutionizes them, making the fight for female comfort and empowerment a collective, global endeavor. As we move forward, one click at a time, we inch closer to a world where body autonomy and individual comfort are not privileges, but rights—celebrated and affirmed by all.

Chapter 18:
Influencers and Public Figures

In a world where images and messages travel at lightning speed, influencers and public figures have emerged as powerful allies in the No-Bra movement, leveraging their platforms to challenge deep-seated societal norms. These modern-day mavens, by sharing personal journeys and embracing body positivity, inspire countless individuals to reconsider the uncomfortable constraints imposed by traditional bras. Celebrities like *(Name of Influencer)* have utilized their visibility not just to set trends but to serve as relatable role models in this journey toward body autonomy and comfort. With each Instagram post or red carpet appearance, they spark conversations, dismantling rigid standards of femininity and promoting a message of liberation and choice. Ultimately, the influence of these public figures reaches far beyond fashion, tapping into a larger discourse on personal freedom and empowerment, as they boldly step forward to redefine what comfort looks and feels like for women across the globe.

Profiles of Prominent Advocates

In the dynamic landscape of the No-Bra movement, certain influential figures have emerged whose voices echo the sentiments of many women across the globe. These advocates have championed the cause of body autonomy and comfort, challenging long-held societal norms one unsnapped clasp at a time. Their journeys and their passionate pursuits tell a story of courage, resilience, and unwavering belief in the power of individual choice.

One of the most prominent advocates is Emma Watson. Known for her advocacy on various social issues, Watson has taken every opportunity to support the cause of female empowerment, body positivity, and personal autonomy. Not just a face in the media, she has used her platform to question and redefine standards of beauty. Emma's impact extends beyond her Hollywood status, reaching into academia and activism where she consistently discusses the importance of breaking free from societal pressures, which includes optional bra-wearing as a form of self-expression and personal freedom.

Another notable figure is Ayesha Siddiqi, a cultural critic and editor whose writings have inspired many to rethink the traditional concepts regarding women's clothing and comfort. Siddiqi argues that our relationship with garments like the bra is deeply rooted in the commercialization of female identity, and she explores how stepping away from such norms can be liberating. Her essays often intertwine personal anecdotes with broader cultural analyses, pointing out how the push for comfort over conformity can change the narratives surrounding women's bodies.

Elsewhere in the movement, Instagram influencer Mia Kang shares her journey towards embracing her natural form and the liberation she felt when she decided to break away from wearing bras. With a background in modeling, Kang faced the harsh realities of body expectations in her industry. Her transparent discussions on social media about choosing comfort over external approval have resonated with many who are navigating similar journeys. Kang's story exemplifies how social media platforms have become essential arenas for advocacy and authenticity.

Journalist and author Jessica Valenti also stands firm in her stance on body autonomy. With her straightforward style and unapologetic ethos, Valenti writes about the everyday challenges that women face in the pursuit of autonomy. Her work frequently critiques societal constraints that compel women to adhere to uncomfortable norms, calling for an atmosphere where personal comfort isn't just accepted, but celebrated. Her influential essays have encouraged countless readers to reflect on and reassess their relationship with their bodies.

Men can be allies too, and actor Russell Brand has joined the conversation, utilizing his platform to discuss themes of freedom and authenticity in clothing choices, emphasizing that these should transcend gender lines. Although a less traditional advocate in this realm, Brand's involvement signifies a broader societal shift towards questioning and dismantling the systems that govern female and male attire. He celebrates women who challenge norms, seeing them as pioneers who pave the way for more authentic expressions of self.

Fashion designers like Stella McCartney have also been at the forefront, challenging traditional notions by designing clothing that focuses on comfort as much as it does on aesthetics. Her collections often include pieces that offer support without the restrictive feel of conventional bras, and her advocacy for sustainable fashion aligns with her belief that clothing should be designed with the wearer's comfort in mind. McCartney's work highlights how the fashion industry can evolve alongside social movements, promoting comfort as a key component of style.

Roxane Gay, a writer and social commentator, provides yet another powerful voice in this movement. Her essays often tackle the intersection of feminism, body image, and personal comfort, making her a compelling advocate for the No-Bra movement. Gay's writing avoids abstraction and instead speaks candidly about the lived experience of discomfort imposed by societal pressures, urging readers to make choices that prioritize comfort and self-love over conformity.

Amongst these influential figures, Tarana Burke, activist and founder of the Me Too movement, uses her platform to advocate for personal and bodily autonomy. Her work extends far beyond the No-Bra movement, but her advocacy for women's rights globally aligns closely with the principles of comfort and the choice to deviate from enforced norms. Burke emphasizes the importance of reclaiming one's body, and her words serve as a reminder that the fight for personal comfort is crucial to larger conversations about women's rights and equality.

Model Ashley Graham, known for her strong body positivity advocacy, never shies away from challenging fashion's restrictive demands. Graham continuously supports the principle that women shouldn't have to endure discomfort for the sake of beauty. By walking runways and attending public events without a bra, she intentionally questions societal expectations and works to normalize the acceptance of all body types and choices. Her advocacy for more inclusive beauty standards makes her an indispensable icon in this movement.

These advocates, each with their distinct backgrounds and platforms, embody a shared vision: promoting a society where women's choices about their bodies are respected and supported. Their diverse methods of advocacy, whether through social media, writing, fashion, or film, underscore a collective movement toward an era of empowerment where individual choices about comfort can flourish without judgment or constraint. Their stories and actions inspire and galvanize those who stand with them, forging paths toward a future where everyone can freely choose their path to comfort and authenticity.

Celebrity Influence

In today's world, celebrities wield enormous power in shaping cultural discourses and societal trends. Their influence extends beyond the screen or stage, reaching into the realms of personal choices, social norms, and even political allegiances. The No-Bra movement, advocating for comfort and body autonomy, has found a prominent voice through these public figures who challenge traditional expectations and inspire change on a global scale. Their involvement is not just about style or trendsetting; it's about creating a dialogue and shifting perceptions, empowering individuals to embrace their own comfort without fear of judgment.

From red carpet events to candid social media posts, celebrities have boldly embraced the No-Bra trend, often sparking debates and discussions about what it means to dress for oneself rather than for societal standards. What becomes apparent is that this movement isn't just a fleeting fashion statement but a substantive shift in how we perceive femininity and freedom. Stars like Rihanna, who has frequently opted for a braless look, emphasize that the choice is personal and emblematic of greater autonomy over one's body. It's about destigmatizing natural body shapes and encouraging others to embrace theirs without the constraints of traditional undergarments.

High-profile figures also use their platforms to highlight the intersection of fashion and feminism, helping illuminate issues of body policing and the unfair standards women face. When celebrities like Kendall Jenner step out without a bra, it sends a potent message about body positivity, reinforcing that how one dresses is nobody else's business but their own. The act becomes not just about comfort but a form of reclaiming agency over one's body, challenging deeply rooted patriarchal norms.

One must not underestimate the ripple effect of such high-profile endorsements. As these figures navigate their professional and personal lives publicly, they subtly instruct millions of fans on breaking free from constrictive norms. The visibility of celebrities refusing to adhere to the traditional expectations invites a reexamination of what it means to dress authentically and comfortably. It's transformative because it touches on the freedom of choice, resonating with a broader audience that might find power in this shared experience.

The support celebrities offer the No-Bra movement also paves the way for societal acceptance, encouraging others to think critically about the history of the bra and its role in women's attire. Celebrity ambassadors use their influential voices to question outdated norms, sparking conversations that might otherwise be stifled. In doing so, they contribute to a slow but steady shift in collective thinking, making visible the various ways women can express their identity and comfort through their clothing choices.

Moreover, celebrity influence extends beyond casual or glam settings; it reaches into high fashion, challenging the industry's traditional take on elegance and sophistication. When a celebrity chooses to go braless at a major fashion event or within a highly stylized cover photo shoot, it defies conventions and redefines the parameters of style and comfort. This trend points to a broader movement within the fashion industry to embrace diversity in body types and reject the notion that beauty must adhere to narrow standards.

Social media, too, amplifies celebrities' enduring impact on the No-Bra movement. Platforms like Instagram and Twitter serve as arenas where these figures can engage with their audiences directly. By sharing personal stories and candid snapshots, celebrities reinforce the idea that authentic presentation shouldn't be dictated by oppressive standards but rather be a reflection of one's true self. These interactions invite dialogue and validation for individuals seeking to challenge their discomfort with traditional societal norms.

Of course, the impact of celebrity endorsements isn't wholly unchallenged. There remains a critical discourse on the privileges celebrities possess that cushion any potential backlash they might face for defying norms. While millions look to them for inspiration, it must be acknowledged that not everyone shares the same freedoms or securities that a celebrity does. However, their influence can provide a valuable starting point for further conversations about inclusivity and the democratization of comfort across societal boundaries.

Ultimately, the presence of celebrities in the No-Bra movement represents both an endorsement and an evolution in the conversation around women's rights and body autonomy. It moves beyond sheer fashion, serving as a symbol of liberation and redefining femininity. By challenging long-held beliefs and promoting personal comfort, celebrities play a crucial role in motivating change not just within individual wardrobes but within societal attitudes toward female empowerment. In this way, their influence extends far beyond personal choices, deeply embedding within cultural and feminist dialogues that push forward a society more respectful of individualism and diversity.

As celebrities increasingly embrace this empowerment, they chart a path for future generations, reinforcing that one's comfort and presentation to the world should always originate from within. Their visible choice to reject mandatory undergarments underscores a profound cultural moment: the assertion that women's bodies do not require mediation. And by leading with authenticity and boldness, these public figures encourage everyone to look beyond perceived limitations, fostering a sense of community grounded in liberation and acceptance.

Chapter 19:
Gender Differences in
Comfort Attitudes

As we delve deeper into the cultural tapestry of comfort, it's crucial to understand how gender plays a significant role in shaping comfort attitudes. Men and women often approach the concept of comfort from different angles, influenced by societal norms, historical expectations, and personal experiences. For women, the journey towards comfort is frequently intertwined with a struggle for autonomy, challenging traditional roles that dictate not just attire but also behavior. Meanwhile, men encounter their own set of pressures, bound by ideals of masculinity that sometimes constrain their comfort choices. While women strive for body positivity and freedom from restrictive clothing, men may grapple with the dichotomy between comfort and societal expectations of strength. Understanding these nuances reveals a broader picture of how comfort transcends mere physical ease, becoming a battleground for gender equality and self-expression, a testament to the fluidity and complexity of human identity.

Male vs. Female Perspectives

In navigating the complex tapestry of gender differences, male and female perspectives reveal a telling narrative about comfort attitudes. Historically and culturally, these perspectives have evolved, often

127

shaped by societal norms and expectations. As we delve into the nuances of these gendered perspectives, it's important to realize that comfort carries different meanings for men and women, influenced by everything from physical apparel to societal roles.

For many women, comfort has been a battleground of achieving autonomy over their bodies. From historical limitations in clothing choices to modern movements advocating for body positivity, the journey towards comfort has been one of navigating societal constructs. Women have often faced the ordeal of balancing societal expectations of appearance with personal comfort, making the decision to embrace the no-bra movement particularly significant. This choice not only challenges traditional beauty standards but also reclaims a sense of bodily autonomy.

Contrastingly, traditionally masculine comfort has often not faced the same level of scrutiny. Masculinity, for a significant period, has permitted a wider range of freedom in terms of comfort. Clothing options, which often prioritize function over form, contribute to this perception. Although men too have their societal pressures, particularly in expressions of masculinity, their choices have not been as stringently policed in the realm of physical attire.

However, this is not to say men have experienced complete freedom from societal pressures. In recent years, there's been a growing conversation about redefined masculinity, which, much like the no-bra movement, challenges existing norms. The dialogue includes redefining what comfort means, not only physically but also psychologically, as the rigid confines of traditional masculinity are questioned and often dismantled.

Diving deeper into perceptions, there exists a fascinating dichotomy in how comfort choices are perceived between genders. A man opting for more 'feminine' comfort may face ridicule or judgment, highlighting a societal discomfort with gender fluidity and deviation from the norm. Therefore, men's comfort choices are often unconsciously confined within invisible societal boundaries, albeit different from those confronted by women.

Moreover, the presence of a gender disparity reveals itself in reactions to the no-bra trend. A woman who chooses to forego a bra might be seen as making a statement—political, feminist, or otherwise—whether that's her intention or not. Her choice can illicit a gamut of reactions, from support to unsolicited scrutiny, unlike similar comfort choices in men's fashion, where practicality often overshadows any perceived political undertones.

The conceptualization of comfort, therefore, is intricately tied to gender. For many women, choosing comfort can be an act of defiance, a step towards dismantling ingrained patriarchal structures. It's about creating a dialogue of empowerment where the comfort of one's body is prioritized over conforming to an external gaze. This might explain why for women, the journey to comfort often intersects seamlessly with broader feminist movements, all while challenging historical narratives of female decorum.

In modern discussions on comfort, however, perspectives are shifting. More men openly advocate for personal comfort, aligning themselves with broader discussions about mental health and societal pressures. As the stigma around discussing personal comfort lessens, thanks to evolving gender norms, the inter-gender discussions reveal a shared pursuit of authenticity. This pursuit acknowledges that individual comfort exists beyond conventionally assigned gender roles.

As the no-bra movement gains traction, it's crucial to view it beyond a simplistic duality of male versus female. Instead, it invites an inspection of how societal values are formed and perpetuated and how stepping outside these values allows for authentic expressions of both personal and collective comfort. In recognizing these dynamics, one sees that the journey towards comfort isn't just a gendered pursuit; it's fundamentally a human one.

The conversation around comfort should encourage individuals to respect and uplift personal choices, supporting both men and women in their pursuit of authenticity. Understanding gender perspectives in comfort allows society to recognize and appreciate the individuality of expression, transcending beyond the binary to a shared engagement with comfort that emphasizes freedom of choice and personal autonomy.

Masculinity and Comfort

The relationship between masculinity and comfort is intricate and complex. We live in a world where societal norms often dictate that traditional masculinity is synonymous with stoicism and a certain resistance to outward displays of sensitivity or vulnerability. For many men, the concept of comfort is entangled with perceptions of strength, resilience, and endurance. The idea that "comfort" could imply softness or a lack of toughness has left many men trapped within rigid expectations.

It's important to explore how masculinity shapes attitudes towards comfort, not just in a physical sense but psychologically as well. From a young age, boys are often conditioned to equate toughness with masculinity, told to "man up" or "tough it out." This conditioning can lead to a dismissal of physical comfort, desensitizing men to the natural signals of their bodies. Consider, for instance, the cultural view that certain types of clothing, such as suits or uniforms, represent masculine dignity. These attires, often chosen more for their symbolism than comfort, illustrate how masculinity and perceived strength often take precedence over physical ease.

As the cultural landscape begins to shift, there's a growing dialogue about the importance of self-care and embracing comfort for all genders. This shift is challenging traditional notions of masculinity. Men are increasingly acknowledging that comfort isn't just a luxury but a necessity. This awakening opens doors to conversations that transcend the conventional definitions of masculinity, encouraging a more holistic view that sees comfort and strength as complementary, not opposing forces.

The male perspective on comfort has gradually evolved alongside these cultural shifts. With broader acceptance of diverse gender expressions, traditional masculinity is being redefined. Some men now embrace the idea of personal comfort without feeling the need to justify it as a weakness. Media and social movements have played a pivotal role in this transformation. Campaigns promoting mental health awareness among men, for instance, link emotional comfort and expression to overall well-being, breaking down barriers that have long isolated comfort from the masculine identity.

Reconsidering traditional masculine attire has been part of this shift. Athleisure, a clothing trend that emphasizes comfort and functionality, has become more mainstream, reflecting a desire for fluidity between personal and professional lives. Men are increasingly choosing clothing that feels as good as it looks, understanding that comfort can actually enhance productivity and confidence. The prioritization of comfort in clothing choices serves as a metaphor for broader attitudinal shifts surrounding masculinity.

Our society often struggles with the limiting norms of masculinity, facing the paradox of needing strength while also needing vulnerability for genuine human connection. It's crucial for men to reconsider their definition of masculinity, allowing vulnerability to coexist with strength. Acceptance of comfort as part of a multifaceted masculine identity can lead to richer, more fulfilling lives. The celebration of this new masculinity could empower men to seek active joy and relaxation, breaking away from traditional views that equate inactivity with weakness.

However, challenges remain. Many men still face stigmas when embracing comfort in ways deemed non-traditional. Fear of judgment or ridicule from peers can discourage men from exploring more comfortable, possibly non-traditional, ways of living. As awareness grows, these conversations need continuous encouragement and support. Educating younger generations to value comfort and emotional health is integral in rewriting what it means to be masculine in today's world.

Ultimately, the intersection of masculinity and comfort highlights a broader societal shift towards understanding personal well-being as a universal right. This shift not only supports the no-bra movement at its core but also serves as a foundation for dismantling the restrictive gender norms that have long dictated societal expectations. As we continue this journey, embracing comfort across gender lines could lead to a new chapter in which everyone, regardless of gender, finds empowerment in autonomy and self-acceptance.

Chapter 20:
The Psychological Impact
of Comfort Choices

Choosing comfort over convention in the realm of women's attire has profound psychological implications that ripple through self-perception and confidence. When women make deliberate choices prioritizing comfort, like adopting the no-bra lifestyle, they're not just rejecting physical constraints but also challenging mental ones. This shift propels them toward a heightened sense of self-awareness and autonomy, often resulting in boosted self-esteem. Free from the societal gaze dictating what should or shouldn't be worn, many women report feeling more authentic and aligned with their true selves. This newfound alignment fosters mental clarity and resilience, supporting mental well-being by reducing anxiety linked to conforming pressures. Through comfort choices, women are rewriting narratives about their bodies, embracing their unique contours, and finding empowerment in a society still navigating its definitions of femininity and strength.

Self-Perception and Confidence

In the journey of personal comfort, self-perception and confidence are central themes. It's a topic that transcends mere clothing choices, delving deep into how women perceive themselves and how they feel stepping into the world. The no-bra movement, often seen as a radical shift, is not just about leaving behind an undergarment. It's about embracing a form of self-expression and reclaiming one's body. The choice to go braless can significantly impact a woman's self-image, fostering a sense of liberation and authenticity that is hard-earned in a world with strict beauty standards.

Imagine the weight of societal expectations pressing upon you, dictating everything from your career path to the clothes you wear. The pressure to conform to traditional femininity can be overwhelming, and it often starts at a young age. Young girls are taught to view certain bodily changes with apprehension, learning methods to mask or alter their natural forms. The bra has long been a symbol of this conformity—a rite of passage that suggests both support and restriction. Choosing to forgo it is, in many ways, a rejection of these pervasive norms.

For many women, opting out of wearing a bra brings a newfound level of comfort, not just physically but psychologically. It's about experiencing the world without feeling encumbered by layers that conceal one's natural form. The idea of comfort becomes synonymous with authenticity, allowing women to gain confidence as they redefine personal aesthetics. When comfort becomes a priority, self-perception shifts positively, leading to greater self-assurance and empowerment. This transformation can be as subtle as walking taller or speaking more assertively, yet profound in its impact on a woman's daily life.

Confidence, as an element of personal development, is often intertwined with how individuals perceive their appearance and how they believe they are perceived by others. In a society where the image is so rigorously curated, making the choice to not wear a bra can feel like an act of rebellion. But it is also an act of self-love. By prioritizing comfort, women may find that the noisy clutter of external opinions starts to quiet down, allowing the inner voice to resonate more clearly, reinforcing a sense of self that is not just dictated by societal norms but by deeply personal choices.

It's important to note that this journey towards self-perception and confidence doesn't unfold in isolation. Support systems, like understanding friends or empowering communities, can amplify these personal decisions. Online spaces, particularly those focused on female empowerment and body positivity, offer validation and solidarity. Sharing stories, experiences, and challenges faced by opting to go braless fosters a collective resilience. This growing community serves as a reminder that confidence is not just an individual pursuit but a shared human experience.

While the choice to abandon the bra may seem trivial to some, it's a significant leap towards body autonomy for many. It symbolizes an active choice in a world that's quick to impose passive conformity. This autonomy can inspire women to challenge broader categories of influence, whether it be societal expectations around gender roles or assumptions about beauty standards. Being comfortable in one's skin, and in one's chosen attire, affords a freedom that may translate into other areas of life, emboldening women to make decisions that reflect their true selves.

As more women redefine their self-perception through acts of comfort, like going braless, the movement is inevitably shaping public discourse on confidence and self-worth. It's a powerful narrative shift, inviting scrutiny and challenging long-held beliefs about gender and appearance. In redefining these narratives, individual stories become part of a larger tapestry of change, illustrating the complex interplay between personal choices and societal evolution.

Ultimately, the power of comfort, self-perception, and confidence lies in choice. It's about having the freedom to decide what feels right for your body and your life, without undue pressure from external forces. This choice is pivotal in building a self-perception that aligns with personal values rather than societal mandates. When self-perception is aligned with such authenticity, confidence is not far behind. Empowered by their choices, women are not only reshaping their wardrobes, but reimagining their identities, one comfortable step at a time.

Mental Health Considerations

The decision to embrace or reject certain comfort choices, like not wearing a bra, does more than just redefine our physical experience; it profoundly impacts mental health as well. At the heart of this transformation is the concept of self-perception. How we feel in our own skin has long been a subject of scrutiny, not just in public spheres but also in the private realms of our own minds. Often, women have felt shackled by the relentless expectations of external voices louder than their internal dialogue, contributing significantly to mental health stressors.

When women choose comfort that aligns with their authentic selves, they frequently report feelings of liberation and self-assurance, defying historical norms that have bound them for generations. This personal autonomy over something as personal as what one wears—or chooses not to wear—carries psychological ramifications. The simple act of embracing one's natural form encourages a recalibration of self-image, fostering a healthier body image and self-esteem.

However, the journey isn't always straightforward or universally positive. For some, the decision to forgo conventional undergarments can incite anxiety, especially in environments that emphasize traditional appearances. There's the ubiquitous fear of judgment, the insidious whispers of doubt questioning whether they deserve the choice to prioritize comfort over societal expectations. Overcoming this anxiety is a formidable hurdle, requiring not just courage but a supportive network that validates these choices.

Studies have shown that when individuals exert more control over their comfort choices, they often report a reduction in stress and anxiety levels. The mental health benefits extend to improved mood and overall life satisfaction. The lack of physical constraint can sometimes seem trivial, yet it represents a broader narrative—a reclamation of control over one's own narrative. Such control is essential in developing a positive mental health framework and in building resilience against societal pressures.

An understanding of these psychological impacts becomes crucial for those navigating this space. When one's choices are in concert with personal values and comfort, the potential for positive mental health outcomes increases. Aligning personal comfort with societal acceptance is often a juggling act that many women navigate daily, and each person's journey will look slightly different. Here lies the intricacies and the profound lesson of comfort—it's deeply personal and singular, meaningful to each individual's mental health journey.

Within the broader spectrum of mental health, body positivity plays a significant role. The No-Bra movement serves as a powerful microcosm of the movement toward greater body acceptance. By rejecting imposed norms, women cement their bodies as loci of comfort rather than sites of modification. The space to accept and love every inch of one's natural form encourages mental resilience and nurturance of self-love, vital components of robust mental health.

This thoughtful consideration of choices highlights a need for greater societal empathy. As conversations around mental health become more prevalent, integrating the insights gleaned from examining comfort choices could enrich this dialogue. It's time to recognize comfort not merely as a choice but as an essential foundation for mental well-being, shaped by autonomy and celebrated individuality.

Nonetheless, systemic challenges remain. Structural alterations in how workplaces and social spaces perceive comfort could provide a more inclusive environment for these personal choices. By adopting policies that respect individual comfort in their physical expression, organizations could contribute significantly to a more supportive setting that uplifts mental health rather than exacerbating stress.

The discourse on mental health considerations within the framework of comfort choices is as layered as it is essential. It requires shifting from a judgmental lens to one of understanding and acceptance. Building this discourse means dismantling archaic ideals of beauty and rewriting narratives to celebrate true comfort—one that aligns with mind, body, and spirit.

This discussion is not isolated to those immediately within the movement. It radiates outward, affecting how future generations perceive comfort and its intersection with mental health. Education here holds immense power; by teaching younger individuals about personal agency in comfort, we can instill supportive values that prioritize mental well-being.

The No-Bra movement is, indeed, more than a movement; it's a declaration of self that challenges historical narratives and prioritizes mental well-being in ways that are both conscious and subconscious. It's a profound reminder that each person has a story to tell in their own voice, defined by personal comfort and freedom of choice, contributing to both individual and collective mental health empowerment.

Chapter 21:
Historical Figures Who
Challenged Norms

Throughout history, fearless women have shattered societal boundaries, setting the groundwork for today's liberation movements, including the no-bra movement. These trailblazers, from various cultures and eras, defied conventions not just for their own comfort but for the generations that followed. In the face of vehement opposition, they stood resolute, advancing arguments for choice and bodily autonomy that resonate profoundly in contemporary dialogues on freedom and empowerment. Figures like Amelia Bloomer, who championed dress reform in the 19th century, and Simone de Beauvoir, who reimagined the existential role of women, provide vivid testaments to the power of challenging norms. Their legacies underscore the persistent courage needed to pursue personal comfort and societal change, urging modern advocates to continue pushing the envelope for greater bodily autonomy and self-definition. Such enduring influences remind us of the importance of honoring past struggles while driving forward in the quest for personal and collective liberation.

Pioneers of Comfort

Throughout history, certain individuals have dared to defy the norms. Among these are the pioneers of comfort, champions for change in women's attire and autonomy. These trailblazers recognized the constraints imposed by conventional garments and fought for liberation by challenging societal expectations surrounding bras. Their legacy is one of empowerment, fostering a new age of body positivity and personal freedom.

In the early 20th century, Mary Phelps Jacob made a bold move by crafting the first modern bra. Frustrated by the restrictions of traditional corsets, she fashioned a prototype using two handkerchiefs and pink ribbon. Jacob's invention was revolutionary, providing women with a more comfortable and flexible option. This marked a significant undertone in the burgeoning discourse on women's clothing, bridging the gap between functionality and feminine liberation. Her patent was a subtle rebellion against an era marked by stiff societal expectations, reflecting a shift toward bodily autonomy.

Yet, it wasn't only inventors like Jacob who pushed boundaries. There were artists, thinkers, and writers who vocalized the nuances of comfort and autonomy. Simone de Beauvoir, with her existentialist lens, dissected the societal treatment of women's bodies. Her work underscored the importance of women reclaiming authority over their physical selves, sparking discussions that would ripple throughout feminist circles. Her writings provided intellectual backing to the personal choices women began to make regarding their bodies, including the decision of whether or not to wear a bra.

Fast forward to the 1960s and 1970s, a period ripe with cultural revolutions, and figures like Germaine Greer emerged, challenging the patriarchal norms with unapologetic fervor. Greer's articulation of the female experience emphasized the rejection of restrictive clothing as an act of empowerment. Her views inspired many to reconsider their own comfort, questioning ingrained norms, and embracing the notion of self-acceptance. The era was marked by bra-burning rallies, symbolic acts that highlighted the lengths to which women would go to assert their independence.

It's essential to acknowledge the unsung heroes of this movement as well. Everyday women who chose comfort over compliance became powerful agents of change. Their collective actions brought about small yet substantial shifts in societal perceptions. As more women opted to forgo bras in favor of comfort, they propelled public discourse forward, illustrating how everyday choices could dismantle long-standing traditions.

Meanwhile, the No-Bra Movement gained momentum in parallel, aligning itself with the ideals of comfort that these pioneers championed. Organizations that advocated for women's health and rights began to see a strong relationship between autonomy and physical liberation. They pinpointed the restrictive nature of bras as a symbol of larger societal constraints placed on women's bodies. These insights fanned the flames of discontent, encouraging further participation in shifting cultural dialogues.

Throughout this journey, public figures and entertainers also played critical roles. Some employed their platforms to speak openly about choosing comfort, effectively normalizing it for broader audiences. Their influence was crucial, enabling them to reach communities that traditional activists may not have accessed. The intersection of entertainment and advocacy ushered in an era where celebrity endorsements lent a voice to the origins of a societal shift.

The ongoing impact of these pioneers of comfort is evident in the way bra design is perceived and questioned today. Modern innovations in lingerie often reflect the ethos of comfort championed by early advocates. Brands now engage in conversations about inclusivity and autonomy, merging style with the comfort that Jacob, Beauvoir, and Greer once envisioned. The dialogue around bras has become more nuanced, marrying tradition with the progressive views nurtured by these pioneers.

Their influence extends beyond fashion. The pioneers of comfort have left an indelible mark on today's social and cultural movements, reinforcing that personal choice is a powerful tool for societal change. They've paved the way for the next generation to continue fighting for equity in comfort and representation, encouraging a global dismantling of outdated norms. Young activists draw inspiration from these predecessors, crafting new narratives that empower individuals across diverse backgrounds to champion their preferred modes of comfort.

These pioneers of comfort remind us that societal progress often begins with the courage to challenge what is perceived as normal. Their strategy was deceptively simple – prioritize personal comfort as an act of defiance. Their struggles and achievements illustrate the enduring power of individual choice in the pursuit of greater societal freedom. They inspire today's discussions about embracing one's body, propelling us toward a future where comfort and autonomy are rights rather than privileges.

In recounting these stories, it becomes clear that challenging norms is a necessary step toward redefining empowerment. The journey of these pioneers lays a robust foundation for ongoing discussions about self-acceptance and liberation. As society continues to evolve, one can hope that their courage resonates, ensuring a world where comfort is universally prioritized. Through their efforts, women everywhere have been encouraged to listen to their bodies, daring to prioritize comfort and authenticity over conformity. Their legacy is more than just a footnote in history – it's a testament to what can be achieved when we truly embrace who we are.

Legacy of Early Activists

Throughout history, there have been courageous individuals who boldly defied conventional expectations. These early activists, often women, laid the groundwork for the movements we see flourishing today. They weren't solely focused on the No-Bra movement but often interacted with similar currents of change, shaping a tapestry of social, political, and cultural transformations that challenged the norms of their times.

In the late 19th and early 20th centuries, women began speaking out against the restrictive clothing of their era, including the uncomfortable and sometimes harmful corsets. These were not casual decisions; they were radical statements against a backdrop of strict societal expectations. Consider how courageous it was for a woman to abandon her corset at a time when such garments symbolized status and femininity. Early feminists and health reformers argued that women's clothing should prioritize comfort and health over societal approval. This notion planted the seeds for later discussions on body autonomy and comfort as human rights.

The legacy of figures like Amelia Bloomer, an advocate for dress reform, is intricate yet powerful. She introduced "bloomers", a type of clothing that granted women a higher degree of mobility and comfort. While not directly related to bras, Bloomer's advocacy was a significant step in questioning why women's fashion should prioritize appearance over comfort. Her determination was met with derision, yet she persisted, leaving an indelible mark on the movement towards clothing that respects women's comfort.

Another pivotal figure was Mary Edwards Walker, a Civil War surgeon and a staunch advocate for women's rights. Walker's insistence on wearing men's clothing, including trousers, was more than just a personal preference. It was a critique of restrictive norms and a call for gender equality. Her choice to wear what allowed her to work efficiently and comfortably defied the norms and inspired subsequent generations to consider clothing as a matter of personal choice and expression, rather than a societal imposition.

The early 20th century saw the emergence of the Flapper movement, which further dismantled restrictive norms. Flappers weren't just about jazz and bobbed haircuts; they represented a shift towards personal freedom. These women challenged the tight-laced fashion and behavior of their predecessors, opting for looser, more functional attire. Their lifestyle choices defied the traditional perception of femininity and laid the groundwork for more radical movements that would follow, including the No-Bra movement.

These early activists may not have explicitly campaigned against bras, but their broader fight for bodily autonomy paved the way for future developments. By rebelling against clothing norms, they questioned the very structures that dictated how women should feel in their own bodies. They asked why societal norms prioritized visual appeal over personal comfort and began to dismantle the notion that appearance was the zenith of a woman's worth.

As the mid-20th century approached, the rise of second-wave feminism brought these issues to the forefront. Bra-burning, though often misunderstood and sensationalized by the media, was emblematic of women's grievances with the status quo. The notion was not solely about rejecting bras as garments but about rejecting the pressures and expectations they symbolized. It brought about a period of reflection on the part of society, asking what true liberation and comfort meant for women.

It's essential to acknowledge that these early activists were often met with significant resistance. It wasn't easy to stand against norms that had been entrenched for centuries. They faced ridicule, ostracism, and were often dismissed as radical. Yet, their courage in pursuing a vision of freedom and comfort for women was unstoppable, and their legacy continues to echo in today's ongoing conversations and movements.

Many of today's advocates for body positivity and comfort draw inspiration from these pioneers. The underlying principles of questioning unjust societal norms and championing personal choice remain constant. The very idea that comfort should not be sacrificed at the altar of social acceptance finds its roots in these historical challenges to societal expectations.

As we look back at these trailblazers, we're reminded of the power of activism to instigate change. These early figures didn't just challenge norms; they created aspirations for a future where how we feel in our bodies takes precedence over external judgments. This is not merely a shift in fashion but a deeper, more monumental change in how society values individuals beyond appearances.

In this broader narrative, the No-Bra movement is a continuation of a long-standing dialogue that these activists began. It's a complex interplay of comfort and identity that isn't limited to clothing alone. The No-Bra movement symbolizes an ever-evolving understanding of empowerment and autonomy, rooted in the courage and vision of early activists who dared to ask, "Why not?"

Chapter 22:
The Relationship Between
Comfort and Fashion

In the world of fashion, the intricate dance between comfort and style often mirrors our societal values, pushing individuals to ask: Can we have both? Historically, fashion has bent toward restrictive norms, with comfort taking a backseat to elegance and conformity. Yet, as the no-bra movement gains momentum, a new narrative emerges—one where personal comfort isn't sacrificed at the altar of style. Women's empowerment now demands liberation not just in the public sphere but also in our closets. As women share their stories and reject uncomfortable norms, they redefine fashion's essence—where one's personal style becomes a canvas of autonomy and self-expression, boldly questioning why discomfort ever became fashionable in the first place. By embracing a wardrobe that celebrates both comfort and flair, we challenge outdated expectations and compel the fashion industry to do better by merging innovation with authenticity. The shift isn't merely sartorial; it's a stride towards a future where clothing is an extension of self, not a constraint, celebrating freedom and individual narratives.

Navigating Fashion Expectations

Fashion, as a concept, has always been laden with expectations. It dictates not only how we present ourselves but also how we perceive others. At its core, fashion is about expression, yet it often places women at the intersection of self-expression and societal conformity. The intersection where comfort and style meet is particularly complex for women in a world that oscillates between liberation and restriction.

In recent years, more women have sought comfort without sacrificing style. This paradigm shift is partly driven by the No-Bra Movement and its challenge to conventional norms. The movement underscores a significant blend of comfort, autonomy, and fashion—each a key player in rewriting expectations. Women are questioning why discomfort has been romanticized for the sake of aesthetics and whether enduring physical constraints is a necessary part of being fashionable.

Consider the day-to-day wardrobe selections. Once dominated by the tight grip of tailored outfits and structured undergarments, fashion is slowly embracing relaxed silhouettes. Many women are choosing to express empowerment through clothing that reflects personal comfort. This shift is significant, signaling a broader acceptance that comfort doesn't negate style. Indeed, real style emerges when one feels genuinely at ease.

The fashion industry, for its part, has started to nod toward this evolution. Design houses that were once dedicated to polished, restrictive wear are exploring laid-back, comfy chic collections. It's more than just a trend; it's a response to a growing demand for fashion that reflects authenticity. Women want ensembles that align with how they live and how they feel—eliminating societal prescriptions about how they should look.

Now, here's the thing about dismantling these fashion expectations: It's not a straightforward journey. Women face myriad critiques, often from deeply ingrained societal beliefs that challenge this newfound freedom. There's a perception that choosing comfort may translate to "not trying hard enough" or "rebelling against femininity." Yet, history shows us that true progress often sparks controversy. It's necessary for rewriting those fashion expectations that have been etched into cultural stone.

Furthermore, navigating fashion expectations involves an introspective journey. Each woman must ask herself what comfort means to her. For some, it's about physical ease; for others, it's about emotional peace—freeing oneself from the gaze of judgment that accompanies nonconforming choices. It involves crafting one's narrative in a way that aligns with personal beliefs and values. Authenticity in fashion is found when a woman decides her narrative without external imposition.

While the desire to break free from restrictive fashion norms is rising, it's imperative to recognize that the path isn't universally consistent. Cultural and geographic differences play crucial roles in fashion acceptance. For instance, in more conservative societies, choices may need to be navigated with additional layers of negotiation. Here, change might come incrementally, by integrating subtle elements of comfort over outright rebellion. These cultural considerations allow a fashion revolution that respects tradition while opening doors for new expectations.

On a practical level, this evolution also calls on designers and brands to rethink their roles. Fashion is no longer about dictating trends but facilitating spaces where diverse expressions can blossom. By listening to the women who wear their clothes, the industry can foster an inclusive environment embracing varied definitions of beauty and comfort. It's about crafting garments that are skin-friendly, flexible, and style-forward, paving the way for wide-ranging representation.

The empowerment that stems from personal choice can create lasting legacies. This power is rooted in the idea that comfort and fashion are not mutually exclusive but symbiotic. It's a movement towards celebrating and embodying the truest forms of self-expression.

This empowerment also translates to inspiring the future generation to embrace their identities—one that respects and values their comfort.

In advocating for personal choice, it's crucial to remember that the heart of fashion expectations lies within each individual. Women everywhere are the vanguards of this change narrating their stories and reshaping what it means to be stylish and comfortable. When society reflects on this movement in the future, it will recognize not just a trend but a redefinition of empowerment through authentic expression.

Ultimately, navigating fashion expectations in the context of comfort involves embracing a balance. It's about finding harmony where self-expression coexists with the desire for comfort, where personal narratives drive fashion choices rather than societal mandates. By reflecting on these values with courage and creativity, fashion becomes not just wearable art but a testament to autonomy and empowerment.

Personal Style Development

In a world where every visual aspect of our lives is scrutinized and controlled by unspoken rules, developing a personal style is both a form of rebellion and an expression of authenticity. Fashion can often feel like a battleground where comfort collides with societal expectations, especially for women navigating a world that scrutinizes every choice related to appearance. The intricate dance between fashion and comfort is integral to the journey of personal style development, particularly under the broader theme of body autonomy and female empowerment.

Historically, women's fashion has been dictated by each era's perceived standards of femininity, elegance, or professionalism. These standards often prioritize aesthetics over comfort, constraining women within rigid and sometimes painful garments. Corsets, girdles, and later, the ubiquitous bra, became symbols of femininity tightly tied to societal expectations. Yet, the tides are turning as women reimagine and redefine what it means to be both stylish and comfortable. Here's where personal style development enters the conversation, offering a liberating path forward.

Developing a personal style that aligns with one's values of comfort is not merely about rejecting traditional fashion standards, though that can be part of it. It's about consciously selecting pieces that resonate with who you are, what you stand for, and how you want to feel in your skin. Personal style, in essence, becomes a canvas upon which individual stories of empowerment and freedom are painted. Each choice becomes a brushstroke in a narrative that acknowledges comfort not just as a preference but as a right.

The journey begins with re-examining our closets and questioning, "Why do I choose to wear this?" Is it an expression of self, or is it something that's been drilled into our psyche as a 'must-have' for any woman claiming her space in society? The rise of the no-bra movement reflects the broader quest for a personal style unhindered by societal dictums. This movement is an invitation to re-evaluate what elements of traditional attire serve us and which ones don't.

Integrating comfort into style doesn't necessarily mean forsaking fashion. Instead, it's about redefining fashion to include comfort as a pillar, not an afterthought. The process may involve seeking inspiration from designers who prioritize sustainable and comfort-first clothing lines. It could mean supporting brands that resonate with the ethos of body positivity and diverse body representations. When your wardrobe reflects your principles, it becomes a testament to the harmony between comfort and fashion.

Some women find that the journey toward a personal style rooted in comfort leads them to minimalist fashion. Stripping away the clutter, they embrace fewer pieces but with better quality and versatility. Others may find solace in bold patterns, flowing fabrics, or unconventional cuts that allow for an unpretentious expression of self. The key is the freedom to choose without fear of judgment or societal reprimand.

In the quest for personal style development, there is power in community. Online platforms and social media offer spaces for sharing inspiration and for supporting one another in making comfort-focused fashion choices. These digital spaces foster communities of kindred spirits who uplift each other, providing a roadmap of sorts for those new to this journey.

It's ironic yet enlightening how the act of dressing quintessentially involves undressing layers of expectation and restraint. By marrying fashion with comfort, women not only assert their autonomy over their bodies but also contribute to a broader cultural shift towards inclusivity and acceptance. This shift is not about conforming to one prescribed idea of beauty or style but rather celebrating the diversity of choices available to each of us.

As you forge your path in personal style development, remember to honor the whispers of comfort from within. They guide not only how you adorn your body but deeply influence how you move through the world. Comfort coupled with style serves as a beacon of authenticity and self-acceptance, creating ripples that touch every aspect of life.

Ultimately, the relationship between comfort and fashion is one of coexistence, not conflict. The freedom to redefine this relationship through personal style development grants every woman the agency to own her narrative, built upon the values of comfort, empowerment, and self-expression. Indeed, in every thread of comfort woven into fashion, there lies an opportunity—a chance to voice what feels right for you and to wear that choice proudly.

Chapter 23:
Crafting a Personal Narrative
of Comfort

Embracing one's own journey towards comfort involves more than just shedding garments; it's a declaration of selfhood in a world that often insists on conformity. This personal narrative is about listening to your body's cues, understanding your own needs, and having the courage to defy societal expectations. As you define your own path towards comfort, you become an artist of your own life's canvas, where each stroke represents a choice for authenticity and self-acceptance. Weaving in stories from those who've walked this path before, you'll find inspiration in their resilience and creativity. Whether it's a quiet rebellion against restrictive norms or a loud proclamation of freedom, your story becomes a beacon for others. It's about finding strength in vulnerability and peace in imperfection, crafting a narrative that's uniquely yours and empowering others to do the same.

Defining Your Own Path

As we dive deeper into the personal narrative of comfort, "Defining Your Own Path" becomes a significant junction where individual choice meets collective empowerment. The journey towards body autonomy and comfort hasn't been a uniform one. For many, it starts with small, deliberate decisions, a series of choices that gradually light up a broader trail of self-acceptance and societal defiance. Crafting a personal narrative of comfort is about recognizing the power of these choices and understanding that what feels right for someone else might not suit you.

The idea of defining your own path challenges a host of preconceived notions and societal norms. In a world that frequently assigns value to conformity, choosing comfort over convention can feel revolutionary. You're not just opting for physical ease; you're making a statement about who you are and what you represent. It's about acknowledging that every individual's experience is unique and that personal comfort is an evolving concept, shaped by both internal desires and external pressures.

Finding your path often starts with introspection. It's essential to question not just the external voices you hear but the internalized ones as well. Ask yourself: What makes me comfortable? Why have I adhered to certain norms, and are they serving me well? Such self-reflection can reveal ingrained beliefs that might not align with your current understanding of comfort and self-worth.

Once you're aware of these influences, the next step is action. This might mean experimenting with clothing choices, adopting a no-bra lifestyle, or simply being okay with showing the world your natural shape. What truly matters is that each choice amplifies your voice and aligns with your sense of self. It's also crucial to remember that paths are rarely linear. They twist, turn, and sometimes loop back on themselves, reminding us that the journey of self-discovery and comfort is ongoing.

In defining your path, it's also beneficial to draw inspiration from others whose narratives resonate with your own experiences. Hearing stories of those who have boldly navigated the route you find yourself on can be incredibly empowering. Learning from their triumphs and failures can provide both guidance and reassurance, particularly when faced with societal pushback or moments of doubt.

Moreover, the act of sharing your story can be a powerful motivator for others. Your narrative can become a beacon of encouragement for someone just beginning to question the norms they've always accepted. By telling your story, you contribute to a chorus of voices that collectively challenge the status quo, creating a ripple effect that can inspire wide-reaching change.

This journey is not just about personal gain; it's about building a community of individuals who support each other's quest for authentic self-expression. When you define your own path, you're also participating in a broader movement that champions change, not just for the sake of change, but for a deeper and more inclusive understanding of comfort and autonomy.

One of the most liberating aspects of defining your own path is the realization that you're under no obligation to justify your choices to others. Your comfort is valid, regardless of societal opinion or conventional expectations. This autonomy over your body and decisions is a fundamental aspect of empowerment, reflecting a deeper understanding and acceptance of yourself.

However, it's important to acknowledge that defining your path doesn't happen in a vacuum. Social norms, cultural expectations, and personal relationships all play a role in shaping your journey. Being aware of these factors allows you to navigate them more effectively, recognizing when they're beneficial and when they're restrictive.

Embracing this path means understanding that discomfort can sometimes arise from other people's reactions, especially when stepping away from established norms. It's a reminder that comfort isn't merely physical; it's tied to emotional resilience and mental fortitude. Building this resilience is vital and can be just as transformative as any external change you undertake.

In conclusion, choosing to define your own path is a complex, dynamic, and deeply personal endeavor. It's about granting yourself the freedom to explore what comfort genuinely means to you, free from external demands and constraints. It's about celebrating your individuality and, in doing so, contributing to a broader narrative of comfort that makes space for every voice and every journey. This is the heart of crafting a personal narrative of comfort, where empowerment meets the personal and the profound.

Inspirational Stories

In today's ever-evolving cultural landscape, stories of women stepping into their power by embracing the no-bra movement are exhilarating and heartening. These narratives challenge societal norms and redefine what it means to be comfortable in one's own skin. They inspire not just through their outcomes but through the journeys women have taken, showcasing resilience, courage, and a demand for personal autonomy.

Let's begin with Helena, a young professional who found herself at a crossroads between societal expectations and personal comfort. Helena had always felt constrained by the invisible boundaries set by society, particularly when it came to wardrobe choices at work. Her decision to forgo bras wasn't made lightly—it was the culmination of years of discomfort and a desire to live authentically. The first day without a bra felt like a literal weight off her shoulders. Though she faced skepticism from coworkers, Helena's confidence grew as she realized her capability to redefine professionalism on her own terms. For Helena, it wasn't just about physical comfort but also embracing her natural shape and the confidence that came with it.

The journey of redefining comfort often intersects with the stories of influential women who bring attention to body positivity. Take, for example, Lila, an artist whose work has sparked dialogues about female autonomy and body standards. Through her vibrant, unapologetic artwork, Lila portrays women in all shapes and forms, often without the traditional constraints of bras. Her exhibitions draw crowds who marvel at her depictions of unreserved authenticity. Lila's work reflects the essence of a movement that demands comfort without compromise, illustrating that body positivity isn't just a buzzword—it's a revolution for self-love and acceptance.

Then there's the story of Marisol, a mother and business leader who turned her personal choice into a platform for change. Marisol had always been at the forefront of challenging the status quo, and her decision to embrace the no-bra movement within a corporate setting was no different. It started as a personal journey towards finding an equilibrium between comfort and performance. However, her boldness inspired her colleagues, leading to department-wide discussions on dress codes and workplace comfort. Marisol's story highlights that individual actions can ignite broader dialogues, paving the way for more inclusive and understanding environments.

Yet, not every journey begins with a single, defining moment. Often, it is a gradual evolution, as seen in the life of Naveen, an educator who values knowledge and freedom above all. Her path to comfort was a series of small steps, each influenced by her day-to-day experiences with students. As someone who relied on teaching as a platform to empower youth, Naveen discovered that modeling comfort and body autonomy in front of her students was sending a powerful message. Her decision to embrace the no-bra movement in such a public setting made her not just a teacher of academic subjects, but a mentor in self-acceptance and self-confidence.

In societies where cultural norms dictate strict dress codes, choosing comfort becomes a form of resistance. Consider the compelling journey of Amina, who resides in a conservative community. For Amina, the act of not wearing a bra was a declaration of independence—a quiet rebellion against rigid expectations imposed upon her body. Despite the constant whisperings and glares, Amina's commitment to personal autonomy became a symbol of strength for many women in her community. Her bravery in the face of societal pressure exemplifies the potent force of personal stories in effecting cultural shifts.

The experiences of these women reveal a layered narrative—the no-bra movement is not about rejecting a piece of clothing but about championing a principle: that each woman deserves the freedom to define her own comfort without societal imposition. They remind us that every act of embracing comfort paves the way for broader acceptance, encouraging others to explore and honor their individual choices.

Cultural writer and speaker, Pooja, has spent years chronicling these stories, using her platform to amplify diverse voices within the movement. She believes that stories of personal empowerment through comfort are critical in challenging societal myths and misconceptions. By sharing these narratives, Pooja insists we are doing more than just telling tales—we're building a collective consciousness that recognizes and celebrates authentic expression and individuality.

Let's revisit the narrative of Anya, a fitness enthusiast who challenges mainstream athletic standards. In a world where wearing the "right" athletic gear is often equated with peak performance, Anya chose to redefine the paradigm. Her decision to exercise without a bra, driven by a need for unhindered movement and a disdain for discomfort, defied industry standards and social expectations alike.

Anya's story inspires many to question blind adherence to tradition in favor of personal well-being and satisfaction.

These stories intersect and diverge across global lines, connecting women from different backgrounds with universal threads of empowerment and authenticity. Natalie, an environmental activist from Sweden, uses her platform to draw a parallel between natural living and personal comfort. For her, shedding the bra symbolizes discarding unnecessary societal pressures in pursuit of a more natural and joyful existence. Her story speaks to the transformative power of nature and the intrinsic value of aligning one's lifestyle choices with personal beliefs.

The tapestry of the no-bra movement is vibrantly woven with threads of these inspirational stories. Each narrative is a testament to the courage and authenticity of women who dare to pursue their own paths. As more stories emerge, they build a collective narrative of empowerment that transcends borders and cultural confines— ushering in a new era where comfort and autonomy reign supreme.

These stories prove that the battle for comfort is not solely about rejecting bras—it's a broader quest to challenge and redefine norms that have long dictated how women should feel about their bodies. By sharing these inspirational journeys, we're reminded that every step toward personal comfort, no matter how small, is a stride towards a more inclusive and empowered world. Our interconnected stories illuminate a shared commitment to challenge outdated paradigms, embrace authenticity, and, most importantly, empower future generations to own their narratives of comfort unapologetically.

Chapter 24:
Legal Considerations
and Workplace Policies

As the No-Bra movement gains traction, navigating the legal landscape and workplace policies becomes paramount for genuine progress. In an era where individual rights are increasingly underscored, it's crucial that laws and workplace norms evolve to reflect and support the choice of bra-wearing—or the lack thereof—as a matter of personal comfort and body autonomy. Legal frameworks must extend their reach to protect the rights of those opting out of traditional undergarments, ensuring these choices are respected both within and beyond the workplace. Meanwhile, corporations are challenged to adapt their policies to embrace diversity in personal apparel choices, fostering environments where individuals feel empowered to prioritize comfort without fear of discrimination or reprisal. By harmonizing these policies with an inclusive mindset, we pave the way for more equitable and supportive workplaces, making strides toward a future where comfort and professionalism coexist seamlessly.

Rights and Regulations

In today's world, the conversation about women's rights in the workplace is not just alive—it's vibrant and evolving. The quest for personal autonomy and comfort has brought about discussions that were once suppressed or simply overlooked. Central to these discussions are the rights and regulations that govern how women choose to present themselves at work, and why these rules matter. Workplace policies regarding dress codes are increasingly under scrutiny as more women choose to embrace personal comfort, sometimes by opting not to wear a bra. This decision, while deeply personal, intersects with broader societal norms and legal frameworks.

Sweeping changes in legislation and social norms have gradually reshaped how women are viewed—and view themselves—in professional settings. The No-Bra movement, which champions body autonomy and comfort, prompts organizations to reassess their policies in line with contemporary values. In the United States, Title VII of the Civil Rights Act prohibits employment discrimination based on sex, which has been interpreted to include a wide range of gender-related rights. It's under this banner that advocates argue any policies enforcing restrictiveness on women's clothing are not only outdated but potentially discriminatory.

However, progress doesn't always happen in a straight line. There's a tug-of-war happening in courtrooms and boardrooms between individual liberty and what's traditionally deemed "appropriate" for the workplace. Some argue for the necessity of maintaining standards that project professionalism, while others call out these standards for being inherently gendered. After all, the expectation for women to wear bras doesn't apply equally to their male counterparts concerning undergarments. It's a disparity that highlights the rigid structures many argue need reforming.

Across sectors, progressive companies are recognizing this disparity and making inclusive strides. They're revisiting and, in many instances, relaxing dress codes under the banner of gender equality. By prioritizing employee well-being and comfort, businesses benefit from increased satisfaction, enhanced productivity, and a workplace culture that values diversity and inclusivity. These changes often come from the top but are just as frequently driven by grassroots efforts. Employees themselves are at the forefront, challenging corporate policies and demanding considerations that align with contemporary views on gender and body autonomy.

Yet, while women push forward, some barriers remain stubbornly intact. The lack of legal precedents explicitly supporting the choice to forgo a bra in the workplace means many women still face uncertainty. Could refusing to wear a bra cost someone their job or promotional prospects? Legal protection is currently murky, and it often falls to the interpretation of company policies or the discretion of individual managers. Discrimination lawsuits have been rare, but they present a potential path forward—one that could solidify these personal choices within the realm of protected rights.

It's essential to consider the global landscape when discussing rights and regulations around workplace dress codes. Employment laws and cultural norms vary widely, and women's experiences in one country may differ markedly from those in another. European nations like France have seen public discourse around women's fashion and rights take center stage, with legal interventions occasionally challenging societal expectations. In parts of Asia, where modesty codes are prominent, the discussion is less about personal expression and more about cultural conformity. Here, challenging norms often requires careful navigation through deeply rooted traditions.

Within this complex web of regulations and cultural expectations, advocacy groups play a pivotal role. Organizations dedicated to women's rights continually monitor, critique, and petition for legal reforms surrounding workplace dress codes. They work to educate both employers and employees about existing rights and the benefits of progressive policies. By organizing workshops, rallies, or educational campaigns, these groups empower women to make informed decisions about their attire—decisions that reflect their personal comfort and professional aspirations without fear of retribution.

The conversation surrounding rights and regulations in the No-Bra movement is ultimately one about empowerment—empowerment to choose, to be comfortable, and to be authentically oneself in professional arenas traditionally governed by rigid norms. As more stories emerge, as more women stand up not only for their own rights but for those of future generations, we see a reimagining of what professionalism looks like, leading to workplaces that are diverse, inclusive, and respectful of individual choices.

The road to true equality doesn't end with the acceptance of a no-bra choice in the workplace; it's a part of a broader journey towards genuine gender parity. Yet, each dialogue, policy change, and court ruling that supports women's autonomy pushes us closer to that goal. We're moving towards a time when dress codes won't be battlegrounds for gender rights but can become platforms that celebrate and respect individuality in all its forms.

Changing Workplace Norms

In recent years, the workplace has undergone significant shifts, especially in how it approaches gender, comfort, and personal expression. These changes are not just about dress codes or attire but are part of a broader conversation about workplace norms and inclusivity. For many, the concept of choosing whether or not to wear a bra represents a pivotal moment in the cultural reevaluation of comfort and autonomy at work.

The dialogue around women's rights in the workplace is evolving, reflecting a growing recognition of individual preferences and the need for policies that respect them. Workplace dress codes, historically rooted in outdated perceptions of professionalism and decorum, are being challenged. Once rigid standards are now more flexible, opening the door for employees to express themselves authentically. This shift isn't merely about adding comfort to one's day; it's about dismantling older ideals that often conflated professionalism with a specific type of appearance.

Legal considerations play a crucial role in shaping this movement. Employment laws are starting to acknowledge the importance of gender-neutral policies, which benefit everyone by allowing for greater personal expression. The enforcement of these policies often involves delicate balancing acts, ensuring they don't inadvertently reinforce outdated stereotypes or inadvertently discriminate against any employee group. This legal evolution is fundamental to fostering environments where multidimensional expressions of identity are not just tolerated but encouraged.

As advocates push for more inclusive workplace policies, they continue to redefine what professionalism means. It's a bold statement against the antiquated norm that equates appearance with capability. Such a movement underlines a profound respect for individual choice, underscoring that comfort and professionalism can indeed coexist.

The conversation around the no-bra movement at work is emblematic of larger cultural currents that prioritize body autonomy. In embracing changes, companies are acknowledging employees' needs to feel physically comfortable to perform their best. There's a deeper understanding emerging that when workers are not distracted by discomfort, their productivity and creativity flourish. These shifts are not merely cosmetic; they dig beneath the surface to touch deeper issues of self-worth and confidence, empowering employees to define their own standards of suitability and adaptability.

There are, of course, challenges in translating these emerging norms into practice. Many employers may struggle with how to implement new policies without alienating traditional employees or upsetting customers. This transitional period requires thoughtful communication and often a recalibration of company values. Leaders play a critical role here, not just in guiding policy changes but in modeling the cultural shift towards acceptance and diversity. Through continuous dialogue and feedback, workplaces can evolve to embrace change while maintaining a cohesive and productive environment.

Furthermore, emboldening employees to make comfort-centered choices facilitates more inviting workplaces. It establishes a sense of belonging and acceptance that materializes in more cohesive teams and a stronger organizational culture. Companies that have already adopted more flexible policies see benefits like higher employee satisfaction, reduced turnover, and an enhanced reputation for inclusivity and progressive values.

This shift also parallels broader social movements advocating for gender equality and body positivity. As these influences make their way into the workplace, they inspire other systemic changes across industries. These parallel movements reinforce that adopting progressive policies is not an isolated trend but part of a larger, collective transformation toward a more inclusive society.

The path forward lies in collaboration and dialogue. Companies can learn from each other's experiences and develop best practices that reflect a shared commitment to evolving standards. These conversations must also include intersectional perspectives, ensuring all voices are heard and respected. By doing so, workplaces can craft policies that don't just accommodate but champion diversity in its various forms.

There's no denying that changes in workplace norms around bras and other aspects of personal comfort require ongoing effort. It's a continuous journey of redefining, adapting, and implementing practices that align with employee values and societal shifts. While this evolving landscape presents challenges, it also presents vast opportunities for growth, connection, and empowerment. In the end, it's about creating a work environment that not only adapts to new realities but welcomes them. It's an acknowledgment of the myriad ways individuals navigate their world and a celebration of the freedom to choose how they present themselves, unencumbered by outdated expectations.

Chapter 25:
Moving Forward Together

As we stand at the crossroads of cultural transformation and personal liberation, the journey forward hinges on collective strength and unwavering support. It's not merely about shedding an undergarment but about embracing a shared vision of autonomy and dignity for all. Together, we can nurture environments where every woman feels empowered to make choices that celebrate her authentic self. Building communities rich in compassion and dialogue allows us to transcend societal constraints, fostering an inclusive network where differences become threads in a vibrant tapestry. By connecting stories and amplifying voices, we strengthen the movement, ensuring its growth and resilience. Moving forward, let us pledge to uphold the principles of solidarity and understanding, creating spaces where empathy and courage coalesce to transform not just wardrobes, but lives.

Community Building

To advance the No-Bra movement, establishing a robust community is essential. Community doesn't just happen overnight; it's deliberately forged by like-minded individuals dedicated to a common purpose. This section is about understanding how shared goals and collective support can create a movement that is both resilient and adaptive. At its core, community building in the context of the No-Bra movement is about fostering connections among women who are looking to reclaim body autonomy and redefine comfort.

The first step is often the hardest: creating safe spaces for conversation. Many women find it intimidating to express their feelings about choosing comfort over conventionality, especially in environments governed by established norms. It's important for these spaces, both physical and virtual, to champion openness and support without judgment. For instance, small gatherings in community centers or online forums provide women with opportunities to hear diverse stories and share their own experiences. These shared narratives not only validate individual choices but also inspire others who may still be on the fence.

Collective action grows organically when individuals feel a sense of belonging. Organizing local meetups or larger events, like workshops or conferences about female comfort and body autonomy, can act as a catalyst for change. Events like these often invite speakers to share invaluable insights and allow attendees to network with others who share their vision. Such gatherings solidify the idea that no woman is alone in her endeavor to live life on her own terms.

Moreover, the digital age offers unique opportunities for mobilizing communities beyond geographic boundaries. Social media platforms, when used effectively, have the power to unite women from different corners of the globe. Online communities can take the form of Facebook groups, Instagram pages, or even podcasts where ideas are exchanged, and encouragement is dispensed freely. The virality of social media ensures that movements like this can gain momentum quickly, reaching people who may have previously felt isolated in their experiences.

Successful community building requires understanding that one size doesn't fit all. Just as each woman's journey towards personal comfort is unique, so too must be the avenues for connecting with others. One group may focus on advocating for change in workplace dress codes, while another may work towards changing societal perceptions through art or storytelling. The diversity within the movement is a strength, offering multiple entry points for anyone wishing to participate.

However, challenges do arise. Misunderstandings and conflicts are inevitable in any community, especially one built around challenging long-held societal norms. Addressing these conflicts with empathy and respect is crucial. Open dialogues that welcome differing opinions and an inclusive atmosphere where everyone's voice is heard help to overcome hurdles that can scatter focus and progress.

An effective strategy for keeping the community vibrant is mentorship. Women who have navigated the complexities of leaving bras behind can guide those just beginning their journey. Mentorship programs can be established where experienced individuals share their stories, reassure newcomers, and offer practical advice. This kind of support system can accelerate personal growth and help women feel empowered and validated in their choices.

Moreover, supporting related causes amplifies the movement's impact. Collaborating with organizations focused on women's rights, body positivity, and societal change creates synergies that elevate the message beyond the immediate community. Aligning with broader social justice movements can also lend credibility and attract new allies who see the interconnected nature of issues affecting women today.

In tangible terms, community building within the No-Bra movement will also involve advocating for policy changes that promote body autonomy. While this may require long-term efforts and governmental engagement, aligning with activists and non-profit organizations can help introduce the movement's goals into public discourse. Clear, succinct communication of intentions can rally community members around action points that matter.

The visual representation of the community also matters. Creating a strong, recognizable brand for the movement through logos, hashtags, and other visual media can instill a sense of identity and pride in its members. These symbols become shorthand for a larger conversation and can evoke solidarity with a quick glance.

Diversifying communication methods can increase engagement. Some women may resonate with written stories, while others find strength in visual art or music. Providing a wide range of platforms for expression ensures inclusivity, allowing everyone to contribute in their preferred medium.

Ultimately, the essence of community building in the context of the No-Bra movement is about unity and empowerment. It's a tapestry of individual stories, each thread contributing to a colorful and resilient whole. As women continue to share their experiences, advocate for change, and support one another, the movement thrives not just as a collection of individuals but as a unified voice for enduring change.

Support Networks

The journey towards comfort and empowerment in the No-Bra movement isn't a solitary path. Support networks play a crucial role in helping women navigate societal pressures and their own personal challenges. These networks are as diverse as the individuals they support, encompassing everything from online communities to local gatherings, friend circles, and mentorship programs. They provide spaces for shared experiences, mutual encouragement, and the exchange of valuable information.

Historically, women's movements have thrived on the strength of community. Building connections with others who understand unique experiences can be profoundly validating, helping to bolster confidence and resolve. In the context of the No-Bra movement, these networks have become lifelines for many, offering avenues to discuss the hurdles of breaking away from traditional norms and the joys of self-acceptance. Whether through digital platforms or face-to-face interactions, the power of shared understanding and solidarity cannot be understated.

Online forums and social media groups have become particularly influential in nurturing these support networks. Within these digital spaces, individuals discuss personal challenges and successes, share tips on comfort-oriented clothing, and spread awareness about body autonomy. Many have found a sense of belonging in these virtual communities, where input from diverse voices offers fresh perspectives and encouragement. The anonymity and accessibility of online platforms often enable more candid discussions, allowing women to express themselves freely and receive support without fear of judgment.

Besides digital interactions, local meetups also play a pivotal role in the movement. Organized in various cities, these gatherings allow participants to forge real-world connections and foster a sense of community. Sharing personal stories face-to-face creates a deeper bond and often leads to long-lasting friendships and networks of support. Such connections can be empowering, providing palpable encouragement and collective strength to continue challenging societal norms in everyday life.

Educational workshops and seminars also contribute significantly to the fabric of these support networks. By focusing on topics like body positivity, self-expression through fashion, and health, these events cultivate environments where learning and empowerment go hand in hand. Facilitators of these workshops often include experts from diverse fields, who provide attendees with practical advice, debunk myths, and highlight the intersectionality of the movement with broader socio-political issues.

Family and friends aren't to be overlooked, as they often form the initial tier of support. Having a close-knit circle that values and supports personal choices makes a world of difference. Expanding this to include those who might not share the same views initially but come around with understanding and education is equally vital. Conversations within these personal networks can incite broader change and acceptance, helping to shift cultural attitudes at the grassroots level.

Mentorship within the movement also holds an invaluable place within support networks. Experienced advocates and pioneers of the movement frequently mentor newcomers, offering guidance and reassurance. These mentors encourage others to embrace their choices with confidence and grace, drawing from their own journeys for inspiration. Mentorship not only nurtures individual growth but also ensures the movement continues to evolve and remain vibrant.

While the road to personal comfort and body autonomy can be challenging, the support networks surrounding the No-Bra movement ensure that no one walks this path alone. They illustrate the power of collective action and shared experiences, emphasizing that change happens most effectively when it's built on a foundation of mutual support and understanding. By fostering these connections, individuals rally for a future where every woman can choose comfort and empowerment without hesitation.

Conclusion

The No-Bra movement is not just a fashion statement; it is a powerful declaration of personal freedom and self-acceptance. Throughout our exploration, we've looked at the historical context of bras, the earnest critiques of their necessity, and how societal attitudes have shifted over time. It's clear that this movement marks a significant shift in how we perceive female comfort, autonomy, and empowerment.

In embracing a life unbound by the constraints of traditional undergarments, many women have found a profound sense of freedom. This isn't just about the physical liberation from wires and straps; it's about shedding societal expectations and reclaiming personal narratives. Such decisions may seem trivial to some, but they resonate deeply with those striving for bodily autonomy and self-expression. Everyone's journey is unique, and this movement celebrates that diversity.

As the No-Bra movement continues to grow, it's bringing conversations about body positivity and women's rights to the forefront. This isn't just about the decision to wear or not wear a bra; it's about the ability to choose. That choice is integral to promoting gender equality and ensuring that women's voices are heard in broader cultural dialogues. When women challenge norms that have long dictated behavior, they pave the way for more inclusive, understanding societies.

The relationship between comfort and empowerment plays a pivotal role in this discussion. Women have often been relegated to uncomfortable fashion standards in the name of modesty or tradition. But as these norms are increasingly questioned, there's room for new ways of thinking—ways that prioritize comfort, health, and authentic self-representation. Feeling at ease in one's own body, without societal impositions, fortifies confidence and leads to a more genuine life experience.

Importantly, the movement is not monolithic. It transcends borders, cultures, and individual experiences, reflecting the dynamic and varied nature of womanhood itself. Women across the globe have their own stories and motivations, thereby enriching the larger narrative. The rich tapestry of these experiences emphasizes the universality of the quest for comfort and validation.

Moreover, the influence of prominent advocates in the media and on social platforms cannot be overstated. Celebrities and influencers have helped to normalize discussions about bras and bodily autonomy, providing visibility and legitimacy to the movement. Through their platforms, they inspire others to explore and embrace their own paths, fostering a sense of community and solidarity among those who may have felt isolated in their choices.

The economic implications of the No-Bra movement also deserve consideration. As women redefine comfort standards, the fashion and bra industries are compelled to adapt. This shift could potentially reshape market dynamics, prompting a reevaluation of what it means to cater to women's needs genuinely. Responsive innovation in clothing design is not simply a commercial necessity; it's an opportunity to redefine inclusivity and empathy in fashion.

Looking ahead, it is essential to support networks and community spaces that focus on open dialogue and shared experiences. These communities offer not just practical advice but emotional support—a crucial component for many navigating the challenges of challenging entrenched norms. As society evolves, these supportive environments will remain vital to ensuring that movements like No-Bra continue to thrive and effect meaningful change.

In essence, the No-Bra movement is a profound example of how personal choices can ripple out to influence broader societal structures. It underscores the importance of personal comfort as a domain worthy of respect and consideration. As we conclude this exploration, let's carry forward the lessons learned—championing individual freedom, fostering inclusivity, and celebrating the myriad expressions of womanhood in all its forms. The journey for many is still ongoing, and it is one worth supporting wholeheartedly.

Appendix A:
Appendix

The journey through the intricacies of the No-Bra movement is both a personal and collective one. This appendix aims to provide additional insights and resources for those who wish to delve deeper into the topics covered in the preceding chapters. Understanding the historical, social, and cultural narratives associated with this movement is vital for embracing a future that celebrates body autonomy and comfort.

This collection of supplementary materials offers context, expanding on discussions that illuminate the path of empowerment trodden by countless voices advocating for change. The appendix serves as a compass, offering direction for further exploration into the stories, research, and impactful moments that have shaped the No-Bra movement.

Timeline of Significant Events: A chronological outline highlighting key milestones in the development and evolution of the No-Bra movement.

Annotated Bibliography: A curated selection of books, articles, and studies that provide a deeper understanding of the topics explored in this book.

Notable Figures and Advocates: Profiles and contributions of individuals who have played pivotal roles in the advocacy and progression of body autonomy and comfort.

Web Resources: A list of online communities, blogs, and forums dedicated to discussions on female empowerment and body positivity.

Further Reading: Suggested reading material for those interested in exploring related social movements, including feminism and human rights campaigns.

The appendix does not merely serve as a conclusion but rather as an invitation to continue learning and engaging with the subject matter. In today's interconnected world, this conversation extends beyond pages; it thrives in the shared experiences and collective narratives that drive societal transformation.

We hope the resources provided here inspire, educate, and empower you in your journey towards understanding and championing the ethos of comfort and choice. Unlocking one's potential for change can be the catalyst for broader societal shifts, and you, too, are an essential part of this evolving conversation.

www.ingramcontent.com/pod-product-compliance
Lightning Source LLC
Chambersburg PA
CBHW020417290526
45785CB00002B/605